THE HEART PATIENT RECOVERS

Health Services Series

THE HEART PATIENT RECOVERS

Social and Psychological Factors

Sydney H. Croog, Ph.D.

Professor of Behavioral Sciences (Sociology), Department of Behavioral Sciences and Community Health; Department of Psychiatry, University of Connecticut Health Center, Farmington, Conn.

Sol Levine, Ph.D.

University Professor, Boston University; Professor of Social Medicine, Boston University School of Medicine; Chairman, Department of Sociology, Boston University

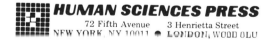 **HUMAN SCIENCES PRESS**

72 Fifth Avenue   3 Henrietta Street

NEW YORK, NY 10011 ● LONDON, WC2D 0LU

Library of Congress Catalog Number 77-608112

ISBN: 0-87705-247-6

Printed in the United States of America
789   987654321

Library of Congress Cataloging in Publication Data

Croog, Sydney H
   The heart patient recovers.

   1. Cardiovascular patient—Rehabilitation. 2. Heart—Infarction. I. Levine, Sol, 1922-   joint author.
II. Title.
RC685.I6C76   362.1'9O6123   77-608112

To Phoebe
and
To Alice

CONTENTS

FOREWORD

There is an urgent need to improve the quality of life for the half million or so patients who each year are discharged from the hospital after a heart attack. A program for return to normal living after a heart attack is an often neglected aspect of the care of the cardiac patient. Such a program should have as its goals early mobilization and prevention of deconditioning in the acute stage and every effort to return the patient to his usual pattern of life. If this could be accomplished more effectively, it would have a major impact on the overt and hidden disability that accompanies virtually every heart attack. This would confer substantial economic, social and human benefits to the patient, his family and the community. It would shorten hospitalization and reduce the need for convalescent care. The present volume by Croog and Levine identifies many of the impediments to a full social, psychological and physical recovery and suggests some necessary remedies.

The rehabilitative process should begin with an assessment of function, not only physical, but social, psychological, and vocational. Physical capacity receives the major attention, but this is not enough, important as it is. Following this assessment it is necessary to introduce programs designed to improve or maintain these functions. The primary care physician needs to assume a more active and central role in this comprehensive rehabilitative process. In order to understand the nature of the problem, the need for such an endeavor and the kind of measures needed he would be well advised to become familiar with the content of this book. Croog and Levine have made a valuable contribution in this field through their systematic empirical study, providing insight based on more than opinion, conjecture, and theory.

While the primary care physician must assume a central role in assuring that the cardiac patient returns to as nearly a normal life as possible, multiple disciplines are required necessitating a team approach. Physicians seldom take the trouble to learn what community resources are available to them to help provide such comprehensive care for their patients. They should become more familiar with them and the community should make them more readily accessible to the physician and his patients. Duplication should be avoided and scarce resources pooled.

To insure success in providing such comprehensive rehabilitative care it would seem necessary to see to it that the ingredients be defined and a structured program of the essential elements designed which promotes greater communication and understanding among the members of the team who must work closely together to achieve their common goal. This care must have continuity, beginning in the hospital, extending through convalescence on into the long-term care back out in the community.

Physicians generally recognize the need for in-hospital rehabilitative measures to avoid deconditioning due to too much bed rest. Physicians no longer subscribe to the classic prolonged immobilization advocated by Sir Thomas Lewis, considered necessary to form a firm myocardial scar. As early as 1952, Levine and Lown began to advocate allowing such patients to sit in an arm chair, advice which was not immediately followed. It is now well recognized that there are distinct liabilities to immobilization which include loss of postural reflexes, reduced exercise tolerance, muscle wasting, psychological disturbances and increased risk of thromboembolic disease, atelectasis and pneumonia. It is now well established that early ambulation does not promote complications of myocardial infarction, shortens the period of hospitalization without risk, and has physical, psychological, economic and social advantages.

This dramatic improvement in the hospital treatment of myocardial infarction which now includes continuous monitoring in CCU's and early mobilization has not been accompanied by equal advances in the convalescent and long-term care. Somehow physicians seem more detached, and less skillful in these phases of cardiac care. Croog and Levine provide suggestions for sharpening these skills.

Convalescent and long-term management after a heart attack are far from trivial problems which should not be neglected by the physician truly concerned about the welfare of his patients. The advantages of decreased duration of immobilization, and briefer hospital stays which have been gained are sometimes lost in the post-hospital rehabilitation. In addition to improving physical endurance, there is an equally important facet of the problem which deserves attention—mental outlook. These are often interrelated problems. Patients and their families require education about their cardiac disease and its management so that they can assume some responsibility for their care, overcome feelings of helplessness, increase confidence and be reassured about their health, family role, recreational and job capabilities. Although the physician may designate the content of the patient's education about his illness, actual implementation of a comprehensive rehabilitation program must fall to a team of nurses, dieticians, social workers, occupational and physical therapists and vocational counselors. Physicians and their patients must have greater access to such resources and they must learn to use them more effectively. The physician and his health team should be prepared to explore with each patient problems they are likely to encounter with family, friends, co-workers, employers and health agencies. This constitutes a challenge to the physician to perform in a more comprehensive fashion than usual.

The problem is not a trivial one. Coronary heart disease afflicts 2.5 million Americans under 65 and one in five men can expect to have a coronary attack before reaching age 60. Not only is this a highly lethal disease, but it also accounts for a third of the disability administered by the Social Security Administration. The wasted human potential resulting from this disease, which often strikes down the breadwinner in the most productive years is appalling. Symptomatic coronary heart disease is an exceedingly common and lethal problem responsible for approximately 675,000 deaths annually and an equal number of survivors. Almost half are medically uncomplicated and excellent candidates for full rehabilitation. In addition, many of the complicated cases improve in the process of recovery so that they too have a favorable rehabilitation potential. Also, a patient who is physiologically uncomplicated may nevertheless suffer psychological and sociological impediments to full rehabilitation. About 40 per cent of those who limit their activities at work do so out of fear rather than actual physical limitations. Approximately a third of patients surviving a myocardial infarction can not carry on their daily activities without provoking cardiac symptoms. They need rehabilitative efforts to improve their capacity to lead a happy and productive life. This entails more than attention to their physical needs.

The Heart Patient Recovers constitutes one of the few long-term reports on the social and psychological aspects of a heart attack, providing valuable information on the breadth of disability including occupational problems. It fills a void in the information available to patients and physicians regarding not only chances of survival and illness in the first critical year of adjustment following a heart attack, but concerning the economic, work, marital and family impact so crucial to full recovery. It provides needed insights into the psychological, social and situational impediments to full recovery. The book is a valuable resource for not only patients and their physicians but for health planners, nurses and other members of the health care team required to cope with this devastating problem.

WILLIAM B. KANNEL, M.D., M.P.H.
Director, Framingham Heart Study

ACKNOWLEDGEMENTS

Because this research involved hundreds of people and extended for a period of years, we owe thanks to a great many persons, and we cannot hope to present a truly adequate listing here. In these pages we will therefore cite only a relative few, trusting that those many others who also contributed to this work will accept our gratitude with the same generosity with which they assisted us.

Our greatest debt, of course, is to the respondents who participated in this study—the heart patients, their wives, and other relatives, and their physicians. To the heart patients in particular we give special acknowledgement, for they provided us with the core information concerning their illness experience, their problems, and their solutions. We thank them for their frankness, their patience, and their generosity in sharing with others some details of the first year after a heart attack.

The completion of the research and the preparation

of the main portion of the book manuscript was carried out through U.S. Public Health Service Grant CD-00068 (Social Factors in the Recovery of Heart Patients). The final version of the manuscript was completed while the senior author held a grant from the Social Security Administration in connection with the development of a follow-up study of the heart patient population (Health Services Use and Life Problems in Chronic Disease SSA Grant 10-P-57537). To these agencies we are grateful for the research support which led to this book and to the articles based on the study.

The research was initiated and carried out at the Harvard University School of Public Health in Boston. It was located first in the Social Science Unit of the Department of Public Health Administration, then in the Department of Behavioral Sciences. In its closing phases the project subsequently moved with the senior author to the University of Connecticut Health Center in Farmington, Connecticut, and the last stages of the manuscript were completed there.

Our colleague and friend, Walter L. Johnson, Ph.D. deserves special note for his important contributions. Dr. Johnson is one of the pioneers in behavioral science research on the post-hospital rehabilitation experience of heart patients. He freely made available to us his interview materials, his counsel, and his moral support during the critical early stages of the project. Though our study developed along a track somewhat different from his, Dr. Johnson's able advice and his previous experience helped us greatly.

The medical aspects of the research were overseen by a succession of three Medical Directors who were associated with the project on a part-time basis. The first, H. Jack Geiger, M.D. played a vital role in the formulation of the medical aspects of the study and in developing cooperation with participating hospitals. His successor, David L. Rabin, M.D. aided in the development of liaisons with participating hospitals, in formulation of the medical criteria for screening patients, and in implementing the study in other ways. The third Medical Director, A. Phillip Connolly, Jr., M.D. served during the major period of case-finding, screening, and data collection. For many months he made the critical decisions, based on medical evidence, as to which patients fit the criteria for inclusion in the study. He also carried out the tasks of coordinating the activities of case-finder physicians in the participating hospitals. Of course, each of these descriptive statements can indicate in only a limited way, the more general contributions which each of the medical directors made to the study as a whole.

The patients were drawn from 26 hospitals in Boston and in Worcester, Massachusetts. A full listing of these institutions appears in Appendix A of this volume. To the personnel of each of these—the administrators, the chiefs of medicine, the medical staffs in particular—we express our appreciation for their cooperation and interest.

The case-finding enterprise in the hospitals was launched initially through the facilitating efforts of two special contributors. These were John H. Knowles, M.D., formerly General Director of Massachusetts General Hospital, and Leon Lezer, M.D., formerly Associate Director of Boston City Hospital. Through their assistance the enlisting of the first two important institutions was carried out, and the case-finding procedures were established.

For advice on the initial research design and then for consultation on statistical procedures, we owe much to Robert B. Reed, Ph.D. of the Department of Biostatistics, Harvard School of Public Health. A friendly critic, he kept us on a conservative course in data analysis. At various phases of the project we also bene-

fited from being able to call upon other statistical consultants in the Department, particularly Jacob Feldman,
Ph.D., and James P. Warram, M.D. Mary New facilitated
our data processing, and numerous others in the
data-processing facility of the Department of Biostatistics
at Harvard aided our work with patience and care.

Over the course of the project we have received
many benefits from the advice of various consultants and
colleagues. In the early stages of development of the
project we were fortunate that in addition to those
already mentioned earlier the following persons were
among those who aided us: the late Samuel A. Levine,
M.D., Bernard Lown, M.D., the late Edward A.
Suchman, Ph.D., Robert H. Hamlin, M.D., William B.
Kannel, M.D., Thomas R. Dawber, M.D., Norman A.
Scotch, Ph.D. and Howard E. Freeman, Ph.D. At various
key points in the development of the research, we prof-
ited also from the counsel and assistance of Eli Shapiro,
M.D., August B. Hollingshead, Ph.D., Jerome K. Myers,
Ph. D., Raymond Forer, Ph.D., Alexander H. Leighton,
M.D., Jane M. Murphy, Ph.D., William A. Claff, David
S. Shapiro, Ph.D., Lenin A. Baler, Ph.D., Meni Kos-
lowsky, Ph.D. and S. Stephen Kegeles, Ph.D. The com-
pletion of the manuscript at the University of Connec-
ticut Health Center was considerably aided by the support and facilitation of Dewitt C. Baldwin, Jr., M.D.,
Charles Jerge, D.D.S., and Howard L. Bailit, D.D.S.,
Ph.D.

A staff of research assistants at Harvard carried out
many critical tasks with diligence and energy. At the
senior level, these were Zifre Lurie, Alberta K. Lipson,
Roberta K. Idelson, Lyn Weiner, and the late Helen
Odence. We wish to note specifically that all persons
familiar with the project will agree with us in regard to
the many ways in which the research benefited from the
outstanding efforts of Ziffie, Roberta, and Alberta over

the years. Other important participants as research assistants were Mary Keegan Brodesky, David Dillon, Allan G. Levine, Joyce K. Hartweg, Jean Lipman-Blumen and Barbara Egg.

The aid of research assistants who helped put the manuscript through its final phases in Connecticut is also gratefully acknowledged: Paul C. Gondek, Edward F. Fitzgerald, Lawrence La Voie, and Virginia Grudzien. To Nancy P. Richards and Hope M. Cinquegrana we offer our special thanks for the care and diligence with which they helped shepherd the manuscript into its printed form.

In addition, there were several other sets of participants who carried out vital tasks, but whose numbers are so great that we are unable to mention them individually here. One such group consisted of the case-finder physicians in the 26 hospitals who reviewed patient records, completed screening forms, and obtained the cooperation of patients and their physicians. Another is the group of 25 social workers who, while serving on a part-time basis, completed the approximate 1600 interviews for the total research project. A third major group consisted of the dozen women who served as coders and who translated the interview data into appropriate form for the computer. To all these our thanks for their efforts and care.

We must, of course, give note to the succession of able secretaries who kept records, typed manuscripts, and performed the multitude of tasks which completion of a research project requires. Among the most capable and effective of these were Ellen Weiner, Henri Turner, Judy Klonoski, Marilyn Glenn, Edna Newmark, and Marion Hughes.

In its various stages of preparation the manuscript benefited from the comments of a series of readers. For their helpful suggestions on the final draft we particularly wish to thank Jerome K. Myers, Ph.D., Raymond Forer, Ph.D., Leo G. Reeder, Ph.D., C. David Jenkins, Ph.D., and Arnold Fieldman, M.D. Cynthia Citron helped us through her able editorial comments on the manuscript.

Finally, we wish to acknowledge also the helpful suggestions which we received from our students in the Department of Behavioral Sciences at the Harvard School of Public Health and at the Johns Hopkins School of Hygiene and Public Health.

This book reports on one segment of data from a larger, ongoing longitudinal study of the heart patient population. Analyses based on other areas of the material may be found in a series of articles, published and forthcoming. Reference to these appears in the bibliography of this volume. In addition, some of these data will also appear as an integral part of a second volume now in preparation—a report on the life careers of the heart patients after a period of years following the initial myocardial infarction.

NOTE TO READERS

This book consists of three sections. The first, or intro-
ductory section, consists of the present orientation
chapter. The second section reports on aspects of the
experience of heart patients during the year in different
dimensions of their lives. Chapter 2 begins the review
with a description of the mortality and morbidity of the
patients during the study period. The chapter is concerned solely with the so-called "medical" variables and
the search for their correlates. Succeeding chapters are
concerned with the "armory of resources" areas, as
exemplified in various social, psychological, and institutional factors. Here we will be reporting on the impact of
the illness upon the patient in each of the principal
areas. In addition, we will review the use of available
resources by the patients. The relative degree of
emphasis on each of these themes will vary between
chapters, given the nature of differences between each
of the resources areas.

Thus we proceed in Chapter 3 with a report on the work experience of patients during the year, and Chapter 4 is concerned with experience in the areas of finances and costs. In Chapter 5 we review the use of resources which are institutional and medical. The succeeding chapter continues with data developed in regard to aspects of the doctor-patient relationship, particularly on matters of medical advice, communication, and compliance. In Chapter 7 we examine the impact of the illness on the family of the patient and consider several features of the family as a resource in recovery and rehabilitation. Chapter 8 centers on the individual patient, reviewing some aspects of personality characteristics as revealed by self-assessment instruments, and reporting on the stability of these personality ratings over the period of time following the initial illness.

The final section of the book is concerned with outcome in two senses: the statuses of the patients at the end of the year, and some general conclusions to be drawn from the study as a whole. Chapter 9 reports in detail on the results of statistical analysis of series of outcome variables and types of association with "antecedent" variables. Chapter 10 reviews the major findings of the report and their larger implications for social science and health practice.

Chapter 1

INTRODUCTION:
BACKGROUND AND GOALS

INTRODUCTION

The episode is familiar, yet always dramatic. In the city a distant siren sounds above the noise of traffic. As it grows steadily louder, people on sidewalks stop and turn in anticipation. Automobiles and trucks slow down, then move to the side of the street. The sound becomes overpowering as an ambulance weaves through the traffic, then speeds by. A few moments later the ambulance halts at the door of a hospital. The attendants rush out, hurrying to remove a figure lying on a stretcher. Doors open, attendants wheel the stretcher into the building and the doors close. The ambulance waits. Inside, figures in white uniforms rush down corridors, converging on the stretcher-borne emergency. The hospitalization and the treatment process have begun.

In twentieth century urban America this is typically the way in which the patient with a heart attack is brought into the hospital. There are some variations, of course. Sometimes it is a police cruiser or a fire department vehicle which speeds to the hospital. Yet for many hundreds of thousands of persons each year, this is the way it begins. To those who have shared in this experience, the life and death aspects are well known.

Some weeks later, another important episode occurs for the heart attack patient, one far less dramatic. The doors of the hospital open again, and the patient passes through, on his way home. Though there may be a group of people, relatives or friends, in attendance, the event lacks the excitement of the ambulance arrival. Few persons not directly associated with the departure turn to watch.

Yet the event itself is of great significance. This patient, as one who has survived, is in a happy and special category. For of those who are sped to the hospital with heart attacks, a relatively high proportion are dead on arrival or die within the first days. For those who survive, however, a series of less spectacular but critical events follow the initial life-and-death crisis. They involve the long processes of adjustment to the disease—the restructuring of the self and the beginning of a new type of life: the life of a person who must deal continually with chronic illness over the years to come.

The patient, on leaving the hospital, is one for whom processes of recovery and rehabilitation are now well under way. While their significance will vary from one individual to another, for many patients these processes may involve complex social and psychological adjustments. They may lead to major changes in life patterns, including those affecting work, family, financial circumstances, and relationships with friends and neighbors. Values and priorities may be changed. The perception of the meaning of life itself may be altered. These processes are ongoing ones, persisting as the patient ages, suffers new illnesses, and evolves new perspectives on the illness, on himself, and on the meaning of his own existence.

It is this episode of departure and its important ongoing effects that are the primary concerns of this book. Each year in the United States alone approximately 1,300,000 persons suffer heart attacks. About half of these return home after a period of hospitalization (NHLI, Task Force on Cardiovascular Rehabilitation, 1974; Smith and Lilienfeld, 1969; Treitel, 1970). In the population at large, furthermore, there are additional millions of people who have been through this experience at least once and who now manage to live with this condition of chronic disease. For example, it has been estimated that about four million people in the United States have a history of heart attack and/or angina pectoris. The toll of disability from this illness can be vast: in a recent year about one-third of the persons who became eligible for disability benefits from the Social Security Administration qualified on the basis of having cardiovascular disease. By any definition, there is a massive and significant number of persons who—after hospitalization—have faced and will face the problems of recovery, rehabilitation, and coping with the condition of chronic heart disease (American Heart Association, 1974).

Given the scope and significance of heart disease, it seems particularly important at this time to move toward developing greater understanding of the process and problems of rehabilitation and recovery. The losses to the nation, as a result of heart disease, have been great, not only in terms of mortality, but also in terms of the disability and the physical and emotional handicaps which affect patients, their families, their employers and society at large. How can men who have suffered a heart attack move towards leading useful and productive lives once again? Answers to this question depend in part on the collection of empirical data in regard to the experiences, problems and prospects of heart patients.

This book reports on one study of the history of men following a first heart attack, their first crisis of serious illness. Covering a period of one year following the initial admission to hospital, it presents a set of empirical data in line with three general aims:

(1) to describe and analyze the life patterns or careers of a study group of heart patients in various principal areas of their lives over the course of a year;

(2) (a) to describe the mortality and morbidity experience of that population of heart patients as of the end of the study year and (b) to examine the possible relationship of social, psychological and medical variables to differential mortality and morbidity;

(3) to examine the variables associated with "outcome" at one year after admission to the hospital, i.e., the factors associated with status or condition of patients in a series of social, psychological, and health dimensions.

Our focus is primarily sociological and psychological. Our method is the examination of data from a survey research field study. But before getting into the statistics and analysis, it would be appropriate to review briefly some of the problems which an individual heart patient may face upon leaving the hospital after treatment for a first heart attack.

AFTER THE HOSPITAL: PROBLEMS OF HEART PATIENTS

What is in prospect for the heart patient as he leaves the hospital to return home? The events and changes which took place in the hospital are but one part of a long-term life process associated with the disease. While the illness experience, in a major sense, is that of the patient alone, in many important ways it also involves other people. The complex adjustments which the patients must make in their lives, the problems which they must face, touch in various ways upon many other persons: wives and husbands, children, other family members, their fellow workers, employers and friends, as well as the professionals in medicine and in agencies and institutions with whom they will have dealings.

Heart patients vary in many respects. The disease afflicts persons of both sexes in all walks of life, of all races and ethnic groups, and from all levels of the social structure. Even where the basic pattern of problems may be similar, individuals will differ in regard to such matters as their recognition of the problems, their ways of handling them, the use they make of resources available to them, and their eventual modes of adjustment. For illustrative purposes, however, we offer a brief sketch of some of the areas where changes and problems occur as the male heart patient proceeds with life following the first hospitalization.

One of these areas is that of work and related concerns. For many patients, questions arise as to how well they are going to be able to perform on the job. For how long will they be able to remain employed? What influence will their condition have upon their future work careers, their chances for promotion, their relationships with fellow employees, supervisors and employers? For some there is a continuing concern that the stresses and strains at work caused the heart attack, and an apprehension that these may lead to a recurrence in the future.

Other related concerns link to feelings of personal competence and to feelings about the meaning of life and the nature of a worthwhile existence. For many men, work is a core activity, one around which their lives are organized. The prospect, therefore, of not being able to perform as in the past raises concerns which are sometimes far more threatening than loss of income. It has ramifications which involve the sense of personal worth, of being a man among men, of the capacity to use the days in worthy activity. Hence, for some men, the possibility of not being able to perform as in the past, of having to cope with oneself as an invalid, may cause them to feel as though they were only a partial person. Even if this were not the case, however, the possibility of a recurrence of the illness and a subsequent loss of competence and control may cause them persisting anxiety.

Family life also may require adjustment. The post-attack aspect of the illness may have serious impact on family members, and the adjustment problems sometimes may be nearly as great or as difficult for them as they are for the patient himself. For some patients, for example, the change is toward a condition of subordination and of chronic invalidism within the family. Since the illness is life-threatening, members of the family may press the patient to alter his way of life, to become a more passive and more dependent person.

In some instances, the experience may strengthen a marriage and lead to an enriching of family relationships, whereas in others the tensions and anxieties provoked by the illness may lead to increased conflict in the home, despair, and disruption. Hostile feelings which some families had been able to sublimate or to ignore in the past may be exacerbated by emotional stresses associated with the illness. The wife, unhappy in marriage, may see release ahead through the husband's illness. Struggles of will between husband and wife, which may have persisted over the years, may become at least partially resolved as the husband suffers the disabilities associated with heart disease.

For the heart patient, as well as for other types of patients who have faced death, the illness may bring about a new consciousness of the self as a mortal being. This recognition of vulnerability may be a critical experience. The prospect of death not as some distant event, but rather as a possible immediate reality may arouse overwhelming anxiety.

A continuing theme of uncertainty will persist over the years. While some may handle this by denial and by a stance of apparent security, for the average patient this uncertainty will be an important feature of his life. He will wonder: Will it happen again? Will I know when it is happening? Will I be in a place where I can get help? What am I doing now that may cause it to happen again? As life progresses, and as patients hear about the illnesses and deaths of members of their family, acquaintances, and public figures, few are able to remain totally free of such concerns.

Often coupled with these issues of psychological response to vulnerability and the recognition of one's own mortality are the hard realities of the experience itself. For most heart patients there are memories of excruciating pain, of decline and loss of consciousness, loss of control, and feelings of helplessness during the attack. Further, many believe that the episode may happen again, and they know of others to whom it has recurred. This is the sword of Damocles: the knowledge that it may all happen again, without warning, anywhere. That one may, in the midst of a happy time, suddenly die. That it could happen at work, on the street, in the bathroom, in bed. The waking at night with pains of indigestion, wondering, is this it? Has it begun again? Few who have not passed through the experience can know its quality and tenor. And those who have may respond in a variety of ways: with anxiety, aggression, depression, or denial.

Another aspect of the long-term recovery and rehabilitation experience is its meaning for religious beliefs and for the patient's sense of relationship with God. With the experience of the heart attack, of having been spared from death, in what ways, if any, do patients change in this area of their lives? In the United States with its heterogeneity of religious groups and sects, with its variation in the population in levels of religious devotion, agnosticism, and atheism, the range of response both in hospital and in the years following the experience can take many forms. For many patients and families, there is immediate gratitude to God for survival. From this point follow such patterns as continued devotion over the years, a reduction or denial of religious interest, in some instance bitterness and resentment at this apparent expression of God's will.

An important element here is that the experience, as far as the religious dimension is concerned, is not the patient's alone. It has meaning for spouse, children, other members of the family, friends, and acquaintances. Ironically, though the area can be noted as one in which important spiritual processes go on, little is known from an empirical standpoint about these processes, their main patterns and variations among patients and their families.

For the heart patient and his family, money and finances are often additional core problems. The impact of the illness on present and future earnings, the cost of the recent care, the possible economic impact of future disability and invalidism—these are matters for which the average citizen typically has more than passing concern. With this illness the prospects of future economic problems come into focus. How will income be affected? Will the house have to be sold? Is there adequate life insurance? Will this affect plans of children to go to college? For many families, these questions are sources of great uncertainty and concern—so great and difficult perhaps, that they may even be denied or set aside instead of being dealt with directly.

The place of the physician in the life of the discharged patient is an immediate and important one. Though the patient may have had minimal contact with physicians before the illness, his life will be altered in terms of his involvement with the medical profession and the health care system. For some, the physician and the hospital will take on special meanings: they will represent, literally, the means through which his life was preserved. Whatever the impact, however, the important new aspect for many patients is the entrance into their lives of a new association: that of physicians and health care professionals in a dependent relationship which will continue until death.

These processes and problems may differ in type and intensity from time to time over the course of the first year after discharge from the hospital. Beyond the heterogeneity and complexity of experience, however, it is possible to see a set of stages through which patients pass in moving toward recovery. One such formulation, growing out of our own research (Idelson et al., 1974), and based on a small series of heart patients, traces changes in one area: that of self-concept over time. For example, while he is in the hospital, the heart patient may see himself as a "fragile survivor," vulnerable to further episodes. After discharge from the hospital, he may pass through a period of ambiguity and conflict—a time of confusion about future roles, of uncertainty about personal competence. This is followed by successive changes, one of which involves the redefinition of himself as "normal," but different from his previous state of "normality." Finally, he may see himself as "a man who once had a heart attack"—a person who recognizes a transition from his former self and is now involved in a way of life in which he integrates illness as part of the new self. This is, of course, but one pattern of progression, and though there are many others, it illustrates another dimension of activity in which heart patients may be involved on an ongoing basis.

These, in sum, are a sampling of common experiences with which the heart patient typically must deal in the months and years following the onset of this chronic illness. This book is concerned with reporting on some aspects of the heart patient recovery and rehabilitation experience. In the next pages we turn to why we carried out the research, our frame of reference, and the context in which its findings can be interpreted.

THE RESEARCH PROBLEM: GOALS AND METHODS

Background and Previous Research

In recent years numerous investigations into the etiology and epidemiology of cardiovascular disorders have been undertaken by workers from a variety of disciplines. The research into etiology has been matched by the vast array of studies aimed toward the development of new therapies and the refinement of current practices. Many efforts are now being made to develop preventive services and health programs which can apply current knowledge and theories to the reduction of the problems of the diseases of the heart (Naughton and Hellerstein, 1973; Rogers and Mohler, 1974; NHLI Task Force on Cardiovascular Rehabilitation, 1974).

Although considerable attention has been given to etiology, epidemiology and treatment of heart disease during the acute phases, there has been relatively less research on the long-term, chronic aspects of this major illness. The recent literature does contain numerous follow-up studies of heart patients which report on return to work, morbidity, and mortality over extended periods. Yet, while these reports have contributed to our knowledge, they have generally been highly focused and limited to several specific aspects of the continuing problems of the disease.

In an earlier article we reviewed some principal directions of research pertaining to the social and psychological aspects of recovery of heart patients (Croog et al., 1968). At the time, there were few published reports on systematic studies of life experiences and adjustments of patient populations following hospitalization for any type of major illness. In the period since then, the situation has not been substantially altered, and it is still rare to find reports of studies in this area (USDHEW, Arteriosclerosis, 1971). Though we will refer to a number of relevant studies at various points in this volume, it will be useful as background to note briefly here some of the common themes and trends in the literature.

Studies of the post-hospital experience of patient populations fall into several major categories in terms of the way they are framed and in terms of the principal variables with which they are concerned. One type of follow-up study is concerned with the post-hospital experience of patient populations in regard to their morbidity and mortality (Beard et al., 1960; Bruce, 1974; Master et al., 1954; Naughton and Hellerstein, 1973; Pell and D'Alonzo, 1964; Sanne, 1973; Weinblatt et al., 1968; Wenger, 1973). The principal effort here may be geared to such goals as developing means of improving prognosis, planning for medical care programs, and evaluating the effects of different therapies. In such studies the dependent variables are usually morbidity and mortality. Customary control variables include age, sex, and marital status, along with medical variables relating to physical status, nature of treatment and course of the illness.

A second category of follow-up studies is concerned with the social performance of former patients, and these tend to focus on return to work and level of work. In studies of heart patients, several clear patterns appear in regard to work, date of return to work, and type of employment. Some findings illustrate ways in which the work potential varies greatly for different categories of heart patients, and how these influence recovery. In addition, investigations indicate that the attitudes of employers toward hiring heart patients, the social class position of the patient, and the work setting all have important effects on the rehabilitation process. Thus, in a report based on a study of men under age 65 who had suffered one cardiac infarct, Sharland notes that men in the lower social classes subsequently changed jobs more commonly than did those from the higher class levels (Sharland, 1964). Pell and D'Alonzo report on a study of male employees of DuPont who had suffered a first myocardial infarction. The proportion of salaried employees who were at work one year later (80 percent) was somewhat higher than that of blue collar employees (70 percent) (Pell and D'Alonzo, 1963). Similarly, Weinblatt, et al., report that 18 months after suffering a first infarct a higher proportion of white collar workers (95 percent) than blue collar workers (85 percent) were employed (Weinblatt et al., 1966). A simple inference from such studies is that the conditions of work of white collar or salaried employees are more conducive to their returning after an infarct than the work conditions of blue collar employees.

A number of studies have reported on patterns of relationships between the level of severity of cardiac disease and rate of return to work. For example, survivors of a first myocardial infarction appear to have a good prognosis in regard to work. On the basis of a recent study of men in New York City who had experienced a first myocardial infarct, Johnson reports that 85 percent had returned to employment by the end of a year after the occurrence of the disease (Johnson, 1966). Crain and Missal studied 184 selected cases of males with myocardial infarct, drawn from medical records of the Eastman Kodak Company. They report that 82 percent returned to work after the illness (Crain and Missal, 1956). Master and Dack, in an early study, found that of those who had experienced a first myocardial infarction, 59 percent returned to work (Master and Dack, 1940). An investigation carried out on 200 cases of myocardial infarction in England reports that variation in return to work is based on the level of severity of the infarct. Only 33 percent of patients who had experienced a severe myocardial infarction returned to work, as compared with 65 percent of those with infarctions which were less severe (Morris, 1959). In the study noted earlier, Weinblatt et al., examined the association of several variables with rate of return to work after onset of the illness and with work status at specified periods after the occurrence of the myocardial infarction. They found, for example, that the proportion of men who returned to work within 18 months was relatively low for the oldest group of men, for those with a clinically severe episode, and for men with the lowest level of overall physical activity at the time of the myocardial infarction (Weinblatt et al., 1966).

In a number of studies of patient follow-up, more extended and deliberate attention is given to the relationship between a broad series of social and psychological characteristics, and varied areas of performance. The list of such studies is not large, however. Moreover, most have been concerned with patients with mental illness rather than those with other types of impairment or chronic condition. In one of the most thorough of these works, Myers and Bean report on a ten-year follow-up of a patient population originally studied by Hollingshead and Redlich (Hollingshead and Redlich, 1959; Myers and Bean, 1968). Their main outcome variables are mental status, economic role performance, and a series of social participation measures, including informal visiting behavior and participation in formal organizations. They report positive association between the social status of the patient, and both his adjustment in the community and his work performance. They also find differences between social classes in the types and patterns of mental impairment. Other studies also link social and psychological adjustment measures to the social characteristics of patients, such as marital status, living arrangements and occupation (Imboden, 1972; Pasamanick et al., 1967). For example, the type of family to which a mental patient returns after hospitalization has been found to be related to his capacity to remain out of the hospital and to other kinds of performance in the community (Freeman and Simmons, 1963).

Research on post-hospital experience of persons with illness other than mental disease has been less frequently undertaken. Some of the reasons for such minimal attention to important dimensions of illnesses and ailments have been reviewed by Sussman (Sussman, 1969). These include the facts that longitudinal studies are costly, treatment agencies may be overly concerned with presenting a favorable public image to maintain financial support, and that there is sometimes a lack of clarity in conceiving major variables. In another assessment which deals with issues in disability and rehabilitation, Nagi points to the need for longitudinal studies that begin at the time of initial impairment (Nagi, 1969). As he notes, most research on recovery or rehabilitation with nonpsychiatric illness deals with a reconstruction of events. Although the longitudinal studies can offset some of the problems inherent in such research with a limited set of antecedent variables, few have been carried out. Some of these few studies remain unpublished.

One important work, as yet unpublished, concerns the experiences of a study population of male and female heart patients, followed for a period of one year (Johnson, 1963, 1966). This study by Walter L. Johnson, similar in a number of respects to our own, deals with a broad series of variables which tap family contexts, doctor-patient relationships, and the economics of the illness experience. It differs from our study in the criteria for selection of the study population and in methods of analysis. Although our research was begun without initial knowledge of the Johnson materials, these subsequently proved useful in aiding the development of instruments and in directing us toward promising areas for further exploration.

In sum, it is an irony of this field that despite the prevalence of non-psychiatric illness of all types, one must look, in the main, primarily to the literature on psychiatric patients for longitudinal studies of social and psychological factors associated with recovery, rehabilitation and adjustment.

Aside from longitudinal investigations, the sociological and psychological literature is replete with studies reporting on aspects of patient experience and on correlates of differing types of behavior with differing outcomes in illness. These consist in part of case studies describing processes or patterns in the patient experience, such as forms of family interaction and adaptation to illness of a member, changes in definition of the sick role over time, and processes of coping with the prospect of death. Typically, these studies deal with small numbers of subjects or cases (Bruhn et al., 1971; Davis, 1954; Farber, 1960; Hackett and Weisman, 1969; Hackett and Cassem, 1973, 1975; Safilios-Rothschild, 1970).

There are also a number of statistical studies which examine the correlates of particular outcomes of illness, including such variables as social status, marital status, family structure, economic resources, age, or specific health services or modes of therapy. The basic methods and variables used in these studies are similar to those employed in investigations of such critical life situations as bereavement, wartime bombings, natural disasters and other traumatic events (Parad, 1965). While these studies provide many useful leads toward which research may be directed, they are heterogeneous in structure, findings, and quality, and as yet do not provide a set of findings which can be readily systematized or tested. In brief, there is little justification for assuming that the level of present knowledge obviates the need for an exploratory approach to the social factors involved in recovery from heart disease.

The problem of etiology of heart disease itself inevitably bears on the issues of recovery, rehabilitation, and illness experience with which this research has been concerned. These complex questions of etiology have been explored in a voluminous set of studies, speculations, and hortatory observations (Beard et al., 1960; Bruhn et al., 1966; Caffrey, 1970; Frank et al., 1966; Friedberg, 1966; Friedman and Rosenman, 1974; Jenkins, 1971; Kannel, 1967; Kannel et al., 1967; Monteiro, 1973; Naughton and Bruhn, 1970; Ostfeld, 1967; Rosenman et al., 1968; Stamler et al., 1960; Wardwell and Bahnson, 1973; Weinblatt et al., 1968; Zohman and Tobis, 1970; Zukel et al., 1959; Werko, 1976). In this field there are periodic reviews of the literature in attempts to evaluate and to build upon previous work. In view of the many comprehensive reviews which have been appearing, there is no need to restate in detail those etiological studies which have pertinence here.

However, some notion of the proliferation of hypotheses in this field is furnished in an excellent paper by Simborg in which he reports that thus far "over 35 individual risk factors" have been implicated in relation to coronary heart disease (Simborg, 1970). These include such medical and behavioral variables as hypercholesterolemia, hypertension, obesity, overweight, and smoking, considerations of life stresses, genetic predispositions, and the presence of a particular behavior pattern of personality organization, among others.

Development of work on etiology is also characterized by the fact that particular schools of thought or collections of effort have emerged, and some of these have adherents whose commitment to a particular thesis has ideological overtones. Nevertheless, the level of knowledge is such that Jenkins recently could remark, "The best combinations of standard 'risk factors' fail to identify most new cases" of coronary disease (Jenkins, 1971).

Among the factors which appear to be associated with risk of clinical coronary disease are a series of social, psychological and behavioral conditions which deserve further scrutiny. As we have indicated earlier, some of these variables which have been implicated as correlates of heart disease are examined in this report in relation to their association with morbidity and to certain performance variables during the study year. Thus, previous work on personality orientation, smoking, and physical exercise provides some useful leads and guidance for some segments of the analysis here. Reference to these specific sources for the orientations appear throughout the text as particular relevant topics are taken up.

In conclusion, despite the scope and volume of previous research, we have little systematic data as yet on the factors which are related to differential patterns of adaptation to cardiovascular diseases. Nor do we know much about the complex factors which affect long-term rehabilitation processes. Few data are reported in the literature, for example, pertaining to the total framework within which patients with heart disease live and the ways in which social, psychological, and situational components are related to the character and quality of their lives. While there are numerous reports containing clinical impressions, theoretical formulations, and hortatory expositions, the volume of empirical research on the social, psychological, and economic aftermath of heart disease is minor. The lack of such studies in this area is especially striking when compared with clinical and epidemiological investigations on etiology and treatment.

Yet it is also apparent that continuing systematic follow-up of patients with heart disease can yield significant rewards: (1) Such studies can provide information which can serve as a basis for more realistic and economic planning of programs of care and rehabilitation in heart disease. (2) They can develop data and generalizations which can be applied both in the investigation and treatment of other serious chronic diseases. (3) The studies which focus upon outcome in illness can also provide data on broader questions of how men deal with immediate crises or with life-threatening situations. Thus, systematic data on the factors associated with patterns of coping with a serious condition, such as heart disease, bear possible relevance for research transcending the illness situation alone.

Aims and Methods of the Research

As we noted earlier, the general aims of the study upon which this report is based can be stated in terms of several basic questions: Over the course of the study year, what happened to the patients in their life careers? What factors were associated with what they were like at the end of the year? These are the core questions. The issue of their health and mortality experience links into both, relating first to the nature of their experience, then to the factors associated with outcome. Before considering each of these questions and how we attempted to answer them, some orientation to our framework and approach is pertinent here.

Sources of Data

Data for this report were derived from a study population of 345 Caucasian males between the ages of 30 and 60 years who suffered a first myocardial infarction. Their clinical course in the hospital was of the "non-complicated" type.[1] Subjects were obtained from a group of 26 hospitals in the areas of Boston and Worcester, Massachusetts. The total period for the interview program extended for two and one-half years, from 1965 to 1967.

Special care was taken to assure the cooperation of a study population whose members had a history clearly without a previous illness crisis of any type. In each of the cooperating hospitals, cases were first screened by a case-finder physician employed by the project. If a subject fulfilled the strict criteria for selection for the study population, permission for an interview was obtained from the patient's physician. A report was then sent by the case-finder physician to the Medical Director of the project, a Board-certified specialist in internal medicine. He made the decision as to whether the subject's history indicated that he had had no major previous illness. He also ascertained whether there was an unequivocal diagnosis of myocardial infarction.

Interviews were carried out in three stages by specially trained interviewers, each of whom held a Master's degree in social work. The first interview took place in the hospital shortly before discharge, or, on the average, approximately 18 days post-infarct. A second interview was conducted about one month after discharge from the hospital. A third interview was carried out approximately one year after the infarct had occurred.[2]

Over the course of the year, the study population was reduced from 345 to 293 subjects because of refusals to participate, geographic mobility, and 13 deaths. Analysis has not revealed any difference between characteristics of participants and nonparticipants which might change the findings reported here.

The first interview was a relatively brief one, designed to engage patients in the study and to develop data which could be easily presented. Patients were encouraged to discuss matters on which they were generally quite ready to respond: how they first noticed symptoms, the means by which they came under care, and the nature of their future plans. The second and third interviews were more lengthy and detailed, covering various aspects of the patient's life, including his compliance with medical advice, work situation, family relationships, social participation and religious behavior.

At the time of the second and third interviews with the patient, his wife was also interviewed. If the patient were unmarried, a close relative was interviewed. Although the instruments duplicate in many respects the questions which were asked of the patients, the spouse interviews also contained their own distinctive items. These questions were structured so as to deal with (a) aspects of the patient's situation upon which he was unable or possibly unwilling to report himself, and (b) with aspects of particular problems as seen from the special perspective of a wife or someone else close to the patient. Other questions covered a number of areas dealing with husband-wife relationships and mutual perceptions.

Table 1. Time Schedule and Outline of Topic Areas

Heart Patient Study Interview Program

	Patient Interview	Spouse or Relative Interview	Physician Questionnaire
T_1	N = 348		
18 Days Post-infarct	Pre-illness Health and Symptoms Denial Work Status and Plans Family Structure Physician Discussion of Illness		
T_2	Patient Interview N = 345	Spouse or Relative Interview N = 306	Physician Questionnaire N = 324
1 1/2-2 Months Post-infarct	Use of Physician and Other Services Work Finances Personal and Social Habits Perceived Etiology of Heart Attack Family and Marriage Religion Pre-illness Stress and Personality Physician Advice and Compliance	Patient Care Perceived Etiology of Heart Attack Patient Health and Progress Use of Services Work Family and Marriage Religion Personality and Stress (Self)	Areas of Advice Therapy Prediction of Patient Limita- tions at 1 year
T_3	Patient Interview N = 293	Spouse or Relative Interview N = 247	Physician Questionnaire N = 269
1 Year Post-infarct	Use of Physician and Other Services Work Finances Personal and Social Habits Perceived Etiology of Heart Attack Family and Marriage Religion Personality (Self and Spouse) Physician Advice and Compliance Rating of Health and Symptoms Sources of Help	Patient Care Perceived Etiology of Heart Attack Patient Health and Progress Use of Services Work Family and Marriage Religion Personality and Stress (Self and Spouse)	Patient Status at 1 Year Appointments Advice, Therapy and Medication Severity of Infarction Patient Adjust- ment

Besides the interview materials, data concerning the patients were also obtained from the physicians who provided care during the course of the study year. Physicians were asked to complete two questionnaires, each coinciding approximately with the time of the second and third interviews with the patient. These centered on such matters as (a) the nature of the instructions given by the physician to the patient in regard to such matters as drug therapy, diet, work, recreation, and other areas and (b) the physician's appraisal of the patient's functional capacity and his prognosis.

Although 26 hospitals were furnishing potential subjects to us, the relative rarity of admission of heart patients with no previous significant illness was a key factor in affecting the length of the data collection period. It required a year and a half to develop a study population of sufficient size for this research. The total data collection period extended for two and one-half years, i.e., from the time of first contact with the first patient to the final contact with the last patient one year after his hospital admission.

In addition to the survey research procedures, a small case study with a selected group of additional patients was carried out. These men and their wives were interviewed in somewhat greater depth than those in the main survey research effort, although the same core interview instruments were used. These materials are reported elsewhere (Idelson et al., 1974), and they serve this present work in indirect ways, such as providing one means of gaining insights and leads which could be examined through the survey research data.

Our brief review of methods of selection and screening of the study population, the interview program, and other features of our research procedure necessarily touch only on the principal points for the general reader. Those interested in greater detail and in technical aspects may wish to turn to Appendix A for a fuller description of our methodological approach.

Orientations and Assumptions

1. A prime characteristic of the men in the study population is that before their first heart attack all had been previously well, i.e., without any significant illness. This special characteristic was chosen as a criterion for inclusion, since it would permit the collection of data on response to a first illness crisis. This crisis of the heart attack is of major dimensions: life-threatening, commonly painful and debilitating. Coming upon men engaged in the full activities of their lives, it transforms them from healthy individuals into persons who for the rest of their days must live with the knowledge of their condition and its potential lethal consequences. Thus, the heart attack has served as one core screening device to study a group of people exposed to a relatively uniform and serious crisis situation, and then to trace their subsequent life history.

2. The study is concerned with the subjects initially because they have been ill. A primary tenet of the analysis, however, is that the heart attack itself is but only one element bearing on the condition of the men a year later. The analysis involves scrutiny of one segment of the life cycle, with the definition of the segment set in time by the fact of the heart attack. As noted earlier, we trace the experiences of the men in various areas of their lives during the course of a year, then examine a series of statuses of the men at the end of that time. During the course of the year the men have been involved in a set of social roles, of which the role of patient is but one. These other roles, such as worker, parent, and husband are interrelated with the patient role. While they influence it, they are influenced by it as well. Further, the

performance of these roles takes place within various social settings and environments, including the work setting, home, religious institutions, hospitals, and doctors' offices.

Hence, the central interest here is the total illness experience, seen not simply as an event occuring at the physiological level, but as part of a series of ongoing physical, social, and psychological relationships. To trace outcome of life experiences of patients at the end of a year, we take the position that an approach to the total life framework of the patients is necessary. This approach is not a new one, of course, but we cite it here as part of the rationale for the analytic decisions which we have made in the development of this work.

This approach to a broad series of aspects of patient experiences is not an easy one. For example, it is obviously impossible to identify and measure all relevant variables. In the analysis we must be selective, dealing primarily with those variables which are within the scope of conceptual and methodological tools available to us as researchers. This approach, therefore, serves as a useful guide in determining the scope and direction of the analysis. It seems appropriate at this point in our knowledge concerning the recovery process, when it is highly questionable whether all the relevant variables have been either identified or properly weighed.

Further, the approach serves to avoid those simplistic interpretations which are all too current in professional and lay circles concerning factors related to recovery or to degree of disability. These include, for example, ascribing level of disability to degree of cardiac damage, or diagnosing cardiac neurosis as related to the availability of pension funds. A broad approach, despite its handicaps, keeps attention on the total range of possible relevant variables and on their empirical testing.

3.   A third aspect of the approach is the use of the

notion of an "armory of resources," or series of supports, as a guide in the selection of relevant variables for analysis. The orientation stems from the common observation that individuals have available to them sets of defenses and support systems which they may employ to cope with life problems. The focus here turns to the positive and constructive side of crisis situations, directing attention to strengths and supports, toward areas which have received less attention than those which are the sources of breakdown, illness, or death. Within a population of heart patients, for example, one may look at positive dimensions. While one can perceive death and disability as sequels to a heart attack, there is also effective coping and survival. The elements which are associated with this surmounting of difficulties are those which may be part of the supports upon which individuals can draw.

In brief, this armory may be visualized as consisting of the total array of social, psychological, and institutional resources which can be summoned in problem situations. Its scope may be seen in terms of three levels of components: a) those pertaining primarily to the individual, such as personality defense mechanisms and physical status, b) those which derive from larger institutional structures, such as the family, church, work situation, and friendship networks, and c) those which exist at the community level and which consist of formal organizational systems, such as hospitals, rehabilitation clinics, and the medical care network as represented by physicians.

To facilitate analysis, the types of resources considered here have been classified into two categories: those which were reported by patients to have been primarily *pre-morbid* and those which are *post-morbid*. The pre-morbid resources as examined in this study consist of those which were present or available before the initial illness.[3] They include such elements as personality defense mechanisms, marital integration, social participation, availability of medical and institutional services, insurance resources, financial competence, flexibility in the job situation, and support from religious beliefs.

The *post-morbid* resources, those present during the one-year period following the heart attack, in many instances constitute a continuation of those present before the heart attack. This is not necessarily universal, however. For example, the supportive wife during the pre-illness period may no longer be helpful after the serious illness, which presents a new set of problems to the patient. Or the wife who was not supportive before the illness may change, and a new relationship may develop in the direction of greater marital cohesion. For these reasons, though there may be continuity, it is desirable to regard the supports in terms of two separate time periods. The degree and manner in which they are continuous is an empirical question for resolution, rather than a premise to be taken on faith or logic.

In the post-morbid period, in addition to continuing resources or supports from the pre-illness time, new resources or supports may be present which were not part of the earlier picture. These include, for example, formal institutional services such as cardiac clinics, and such professionals as physicians, social workers, and visiting nurses. They include also supports which were previously available but which were not used as supports, such as religion, members of the extended family, and neighbors.

The "armory of resources" notion is employed here in keeping with the exploratory approach of this study. It serves as a means of directing attention to a series of areas which may be conceptualized as supports, ranging from physical and psychological to social and institutional. Thus, the idea of armory of resources had its initial importance in the formulation of variables to be included in the present work. These efforts led to the development of a series of indices designed to deal with a number of support areas. From these were culled items which seemed feasible and useful for inclusion in survey research interviews.

It should be clear that in looking at "supports" in relation to outcome, we are centering on statistical relationships, not on the differential meaning of particular supports for individuals. For example, stability in the husband-wife relationship may be correlated with favorable outcome for the patient at the end of one year. However, within a series of stable marriages many types of marital relationships can be found. Individuals may in fact be bound together in a symbiotic dyad of hostility. Since the hostility may be giving satisfaction and emotional release to both, their marriage continues, and it is classified as "stable" on the basis of the criterion of continuity over time. Thus, in a statistical sense, there may be a correlation between favorable outcome at one year and "stable marriage." The underlying components which contribute to stability—and which are part of the support—remain for further research. The survey research method employed here has limitations for dealing with the underlying nuances, although it can point up the possible presence of relationship between broad variables.

This orientation and its related procedures are not new, and they draw upon formulations and methods common in the field. They are linked to the rich line of theoretical development tracing back to Durkheim and to his theories concerning social integration and suicide. From psychoanalysis and psychiatry have come theories concerning personality defense mechanisms. In the less obvious disciplines of military tactics and strategy may be found analogous concerns in conceptualizing the array of resources, support, and defenses. Our procedure here, therefore, is to use the concept as an organizing principle and orientation.

4. In addition to the "armory of resources" concept, a pragmatic principle has guided the selection of variables in this study. Numerous hypotheses have been advanced to explain the etiology of heart disease and the course of the recovery process. These center on such factors as level of physical activity, degree of stress, personality patterns, and such "risk" factors as smoking and cholesterol level. As part of this exploratory effort to review pertinent variables in the total environment, we have freely included items which bear on these current hypotheses.

5. Though the primary focus is upon variables related to recovery and on the experience of patients during the year, issues of etiology of coronary heart disease nonetheless become relevant at several points. For example, some of the variables examined in relation to post-hospital experience may possibly have had an etiological role in the first heart attack. In this report, however, our attention centers entirely on their place in the post-hospital experience.

In Chapter 2 the problem of etiology is most directly pertinent. In that chapter we report on illness experience during the year, and reference is made also to exploration of related variables. There is no assumption that the factors determining the post-hospital illness experience are the same or similar in operation to those of the pre-morbid stage. A variable may indeed have played a role in the etiology of the illness, but its influence during the period after the first myocardial infarction may be of a different order than during the pre-morbid period. Our position is that the complex issue is one for resolution by empirical study, and its resolution is well beyond the sphere of this research.

The procedure in Chapter 2, therefore, is simply to examine some variables in terms of their possible etiological implications in relation to the recovery period. In other words, the effort is directed toward screening those variables which appear to have a statistical relationship to development of illness *subsequent* to the first heart attack. These same variables, however, are also employed in the larger analysis on the natural history of the illness experience and on outcome.

6. Finally, several other important aspects of the analysis must also be made explicit. This study reviews a particular time segment in the lives of the patients, and at the end of the period it is focused upon their statuses in differing areas of their lives. Implications of general "recovery," "adjustment," or "adaptation" are deliberately avoided.

Why have we made the major decision to employ a multi-item system for rating outcome, rather than a single, simple summary? The reasons are many, but the prime one is that we wish to preserve in our ratings some sense of the complex phenomena involved and reference to the varied dimensions which they tap.

To undertake assessments of recovery involves application of a series of value judgments as to the physiological, psychological, and social criteria for recovery. While some may term a man as "recovered" if he is back at work, according to other criteria he may be in a dangerous situation by virtue of his undertaking inappropriate tasks. Depression in a particular heart patient at one year after the heart attack may be rated by some judges as a negative sign, while others may regard it as a response within the "normal" range consistent with his previous personality. Differences in values within subcultural systems of the United States and variations on a cross-national and an historical basis render even more complex the problems of developing criteria for "adjustment," "recovery," or "rehabilitation."

In the analysis, the dependent "status" or "recovery" variables are specified in terms of a series of outcomes in various dimensions of life. These are classified, as later indicated in Chapter 9, as primary and secondary measures, depending upon their degree of generality. Using these variables and others, we deal with the general problem of "recovery" or "rehabilitation" in two principal ways: (1) description of the experience of patients in some principal areas of their lives during the year, including health, work, family relationships, and economic status (2) examination of antecedent variables in relation to each of the "outcome" variables. The latter "outcome" variables are classified in order to serve as operational indices of condition in various areas of life, such as work, emotional status, health status, and others.

PLAN OF ANALYSIS AND REPORTING

With this background information on aims and orientation, we can now turn specifically to a review of the format for analysis of data for this study and of the pattern of presentation in chapters. Although we follow a format for analysis which is relatively standard, it seems useful here to make the procedures explicit. For many readers the discussion will be a familiar description of data analysis methods common in research of this type. Some may therefore wish to skip the next pages of discussion.

First, we present a brief recapitulation. The three primary aims of this study, as we reported them earlier, center on a double task: (1) reporting of the impact of the heart attack upon the lives of the men in various areas, such as physical health, mental status, work, finances, family, and their relationships with their physicians, and (2) examination of variables associated with differing patterns of outcomes or statuses at the end of the year in the various areas of their lives. Underlying the pursuit of these goals are the guiding notions of "armory of resources," providing a context within which we may examine (1) impact and (2) outcomes. It provides one basis for selection of particular areas within which the examination of data can be made, drawing our attention to levels of resources of the individual, institution and community. We employ it also in procedures for analysis—to determine, for example, how elements within resource areas such as the family are related to outcome for the patient over the course of the year.

In line with these aims and this framework, we developed a systematic analysis of data which follows the general framework recorded in the chapter organization of this book. The core analysis areas selected were work, family, financial status, the doctor-patient relationship, physical health resources, personality resources, and others.

A sample listing of items from the T_1 and the T_2 interviews appears in the Appendix, providing an indication of the nature of the line of questioning and the areas of categorization. The T_3 interview reproduced in many respects the format of the T_2 session, and examples are therefore not provided. The actual items are explored in greater detail, of course, in the text of this book and in tables, as we describe findings.

A series of independent variables were examined in relation to a series of dependent variables specific to the particular problem area under examination. These independent variables were of two types: (1) those which formed a core group of independent variables for this study and which were consistently examined in relation to all dependent variables of a major nature, and (2) those which were relevant to the conceptual issue or problem under consideration but which were inappropriate to employ on a general screening basis in the same manner as Type 1.

The core independent variables which were consistently examined in relation to virtually all data were: measures of illness level, social status indicators, educational level and occupational level. Those of Type 2 can be subdivided into (a) those which were of relatively generic use and (b) those which were specific to the conceptual issue at hand. Thus, in the Type 2 kind of dependent variables we are discussing relative degree of specificity. Examples of Category (a) are such variables as age, religion, ethnic origin, and income level. Examples of Category (b) are items such as particular sets of personality characteristics, sets of beliefs concerning the etiology of the heart attack, or presence of a confidant.[4]

Selection of the dependent variables to be examined was determined on the basis of two general principles: (1) the relevance of the information to our purposes of documenting and describing the life patterns or careers of the heart patients, and/or the relevance of the variable to issues in the research literature which were of theoretical or clinical importance. The ways in which both independent variables of various types and the dependent variables were selected and employed in particular analyses can be illustrated with some brief examples relating to work experience.

For instance, in the area of work we first reviewed the data breakdown and distributions on those items which would be useful for reporting on such matters as rate of work return, employment problems, problems at work relating to the heart attack, and job satisfaction before and after hospitalization. We next examined these dependent variables in terms of the major independent variables of Type 1. Guiding these efforts were a series of successive hypotheses framed in similar terms, as far as the dependent variable was concerned. For example, in regard to the variable, "interval between the first hospital admission and date of return to work" we hypothesized "illness level is related to the interval," "educational level of the patient is related to the interval," "occupational level of the patient is related to the interval," and so on.

Based on our review of the relevant literature, we explored also the relationships between date of return work and other variables of special theoretical and/or clinical interest. There is a broad background of hypotheses concerning the role of personality factors in the etiology of the disease and in determining post-hospital performance. With these in mind, we developed some tentative conceptions, such as that men with specified characteristics similar to that of the common coronary personality type (aggressive, ambitious, etc.) would be more likely to return to work sooner than those who were of a more passive, easygoing nature. Hence, a series of personality items (which will be described more fully later in this book) were examined in relation to rate of return to work.

Another widely disseminated conception in this area is the "secondary gain" hypothesis, which may be described in part as holding that the availability of insurance supports is a negative factor in affecting return to work. In other words, men who have various forms of federal, state, or private insurance compensation will have low motivation to return to work. This will be reflected in an association between the availability and use of these funds and rate of return. With this question in mind, we then examined whether there was indeed a relationship between the two variables.

These examples serve as illustration of the program and methods used throughout the data analysis procedures for this book. It should be clear that on some analyses we used a standard format. The nature of the areas under examination differed greatly, however, and the kinds of theoretical or clinical questions associated with each varied. Hence, along with the standard format approach, we carried out sub-studies centering on issues and questions of theoretical and practical concern.

The major portion of the analysis relies upon cross-tabulations of two variables. Where control variables were used, this was done at the level of one control, acceding in part to restrictions imposed by the size of the sub-populations and the need for sufficient numbers in cells. The primary control variables were those which were employed as independent variables of Type 1, as we have noted earlier. These were selected on several primary grounds.

In the initial analytic phases of this study, a series of cross-tabulations were carried out in order to determine which variables were the more effective predictors of "outcome" in various social and psychological dimensions. Among the variables screened, those most consistently related to outcome were indicators of social status, including educational level, occupational level, income. In addition, as expected, indicators of level of illness during the year were also related to outcome. Other variables such as age, marital status, ethnic origin, religion, personality self-rating items, and others were not found to be significant as explanatory of outcome. Hence, given the importance of social status and illness level variables, we have chosen to hold these as the main control variables.

In addition, other conceptual and theoretical influences turned the analysis to these two types of variables. It seemed obvious that patients who were well during the year and those who were subsequently ill should not simply be lumped together for analysis. A general problem in classification of patients by level of illness appeared, however. As we will show later in this report, this was resolved by using as a criterion of illness whether or not the patient had been rehospitalized during the year. While even here the criterion for level of illness is not a perfect one, we do know that the rehospitalized patients differ from those not rehospitalized on the basis of decisions made by medical personnel concerning illness.

Theoretical justification for selection of social status indicators as control variables was also a relatively clear-cut matter. A vast amount of literature now exists pointing up the relationship between social status and a host of variables such as mortality, morbidity, health practices, availability of medical care, educational opportunities, and religious practices.

Use of the two categories as main control variables did not, of course, preclude the use of others, and in this volume we employ other variables as controls wherever it appears that data will be clarified by their use.

In the succeeding chapters, the outcome of this analysis is reported. The chapters contain descriptive data on aspects of the experience of the heart patients in the areas selected for report. They also present reports on data developed in line with the theoretical issues and practical questions which we have chosen to explore on the basis of their currency and importance in the literature. In each chapter the issues and questions are described and we will not list them all in detail at this point.

Because of the non-parametric nature of these data, we have employed the Chi-square test and the gamma score as the main means of testing for significant differences and for relationships. Some few exceptions were made, as in the case of personality data in Chapter 8, where a factor analysis was carried out. The level of significance was set at the .05 level. In interpretation of gamma scores the criterion level was .25.

In a study with a large number of variables with which many cross-tabulations are made, inevitably a number of significant relationships occur by chance. Moreover, because of the size of the study population some statistically significant findings may appear, even though actual differences in proportions between variables are relatively minor. We have therefore taken a conservative approach in reporting and in many instances, though there was "statistical significance," we have chosen not to report the data if there was clearly a lack of conceptual congruity.

In some instances, however, even though there was no statistical significance, we have chosen to point up a series of relationships of special interest. If the findings were in the direction of significance, were consistent, and were directly relevant to a theoretical issue or problem, we chose to report them. This was done on the basis that in a study of this sort one should not screen meaningful findings on statistical grounds alone. This will be evident in particular in Chapter 9, where the findings in direction of significance had greater relevance than elsewhere.

In a data analysis effort of the dimension necessary for this report, inevitably a number of hypotheses, leads, or questions simply do not "pan out." Should we report on each of these—on the initial questions, on the tabulations, on the interpretations, on the negative results? The issue has many sides and is difficult to resolve. However, in the interests of economy of effort and to spare the general reader, we have chosen to report in detail only on those relationships or outcomes of analysis which were meaningful for the issues under examination.

Limitations and Reservations

In association with discussion of the formal aims and purposes of this research, some questions may arise regarding the basis for the particular focus of this study and its potential for generalization. Readers may question, for example, the absence of female heart patients in the study population. Why are there no blacks, Orientals, Puerto Ricans? Given the fact that heart disease is a pervasive illness, why are there these major omissions? If this study deals only with a select group of patients, is it fair to generalize these data to all heart patients? We cannot deal with all major possible questions of this nature in these pages, and hopefully, the goals of this report as a social science study are clear. However, some brief remarks may serve to clarify both the nature of the focus and the rationale for particular omissions and for conservative interpretations.

Heart disease is, indeed, a health problem of major dimensions among the female population. The incidence of the disease among young and middle-aged women is substantially lower, however, than that among men of similar age categories. Bengtsson, reporting on a large scale study in Sweden, points out that the incidence of myocardial infarction was about eight times higher in men than in women in the age groups 54 and younger (Bengtsson, 1973). Similar findings are reported by others in the United States (Dawber et al., 1957; Weinblatt et al., 1973). Since we are concerned in this study with the economically productive years of life and the effects of illness, it seemed appropriate, therefore, to deal with a male population, considering the fact that the illness was of greater prevalence among men than among women. As to developing this as a joint study of men and women together, practical problems of funds, feasibility, manpower, and time restricted us solely to males.

The study population consists solely of white males because of the nature of our medical criteria for inclusion and the nature of the racial and ethnic composition of the Boston and Worcester areas. Briefly put, there were few non-Caucasians who were treated in the hospitals for first myocardial infarction and who fit the criteria of no major previous illnesses. Only a few black men and one Oriental fit the criteria. Given the problems of carrying out a statistical analysis of data with clearly insufficient numbers of non-Caucasians, we made the decision to include only white males in the study group. This decision was one which we would have preferred not to make, since we had originally been looking forward to reporting on the recovery and rehabilitation problems of men of differing racial, social class, and ethnic origins. Hopefully, these purposes will be fulfilled by other investigators in the future.

Additionally, we should like to point out that economic conditions have changed and the course of inflation has continued over recent years. Hence the data on level of employment, income levels, and on opportunities for work available to the heart patients must be evaluated in terms of the period when the data for this study were collected.

Finally, we should like to emphasize again unequivocally, that this report deals with one select, subcategory of heart patients and that our findings cannot be simplistically generalized to all heart patients. As we have pointed out, the study population was selected for a set of particular reasons, among which was our interest in tracing the sequellae of the disease without the confounding effect of other previous ailments. We have been able to report on one group of heart patients in the context of a single major disease. This group is not representative of heart patients in general, however, and caution must be exercised in generalizing beyond this particular study population.

NOTES

1. Patients who developed additional illnesses or syndromes while in the hospital were excluded from the study. Specifically, we have included only those whose course of recovery from first myocardial infarction was "without complications" in the medical sense.
2. In this chapter as well as throughout the volume, several key symbols will be used as designations of the three principal time stages of this study. "T_1" refers to the period in the hospital, approximately three weeks after admission for the first myocardial infarction. "T_2" refers to the period at one month after discharge from the hospital, approximately seven weeks after the admission to the hospital. "T_3" refers to the period one year after the initial hospital admission. It thus designates also the end of the study year. As interviews with the patients were held at the time of T_1, T_2 and T_3, these symbols are also used in the text to refer to the interviews themselves as well as the time period when they occurred.
3. In referring to pre-morbid resources as an analytic tool, we are obviously referring to constructs. These can be differentiated from another set of constructs, post-morbid resources. The methodological issue of definition of pre-morbid resources is another matter, however. On many of these resources, we have clear information. For example, age, sex, ethnic origin, and religion are items on which one can have high confidence concerning patient status before the heart attack. On other matters,

however, we rely on patient information such as retrospective reports on social participation, marital satisfaction, work relationships, etc., as they existed before the heart attack. How these latter type pre-morbid resources are defined is made clear in the text where relevant.

4. Examples of classification and coding of some selected independent and dependent variables are as follows:

(1) Level of illness was classified according to several criteria. One was the criterion of death or rehospitalization during the study year versus non-rehospitalization. A second classification was (a) death or rehospitalization during the study year, (b) no rehospitalization during the study year, but the patient was described by his physician as having developed additional significant disorders associated with arteriosclerotic heart disease, and (c) patient survived the study year, was not rehospitalized, and was not described by his physician in the manner noted in category (b). In other words, no evidence of ill health of the type specified in categories (a) and (b) above was reported. Other variants on this were employed, such as the exclusion of non-heart causes of rehospitalization or non-heart deaths. These are explained in the text. For additional information on criteria and categories, see Chapter 2.

(2) Educational level was coded according to whether the patient had completed one year of college or more, four years of high school, or three years or less of high school.

(3) Four occupational categories were employed based upon the Hollingshead Index of Social Position, 1957. Group 1 = occupational categories 1 and 2 on the Hollingshead scale; Group 2 = categories 3 and 4; Group 3 = category 5; and Group 4 = categories 6 and 7.

(4) Three principal age groups were coded: 30 through 39 years, 40 through 49, and 50 through 60.

(5) For analysis of ethnic origin, five groups were defined: British-Old American, Irish, Italian, Jewish and Mixed. Patients were placed into these categories on the basis of their responses concerning the nationality background or ethnic origin of both parents. Only those patients both of whose parents were identified as of British-Old American, Irish or Italian origins were included in those categories. Patients classified as belonging to the "Jewish" ethnic group were placed in this category on the basis of self-reported religion.

(6) The self-rating personality items were: sense of humor, sense of duty, stubborness, gets angry easily, feelings easily hurt,

nervous or irritable, easygoing, moody, jealous, likes to take responsibility, dominating, critical of others, easily excited, shy, likes belonging to organizations, easily depressed, self-centered, being in a hurry, being ambitious, eating rapidly, being hard driving, and putting a lot of effort into things. Patients or spouses were classified into three categories depending upon whether they characterized themselves as having the trait "Very much" or "Considerably"; "Somewhat" or "A little"; or "Not at all."

For a more complete description of the personality rating scale and its derivation, refer to Chapter 8.

(7) Patients were asked to rate a series of items pertaining to their belief as to the importance of each in contributing to their heart attack. Items were: kind of food they ate, being overweight, working too hard physically, bad luck, being "run-down," tension at work, "will of God," punishment for doing wrong in life, payment for sins, worry, heredity, nerves, smoking, drinking, problems with children, and problems with wife. Ratings were: "Very Important," "Somewhat Important" and "Not Important at All."

(8) The item "presence of a confidant" stems from the question, "Do you feel you have someone to talk with about the really important things on your mind?". Responses were coded according to a simple "yes" or "no" system.

(9) Perceived subjective health level was measured by the number of symptoms associated with heart disease which the patient reported as having experienced during the month previous to the T_3 interview. Categories were as follows: None; Low = one or two; High = three or more. For additional information on symptoms refer to Chapter 9.

Chapter 2

MORBIDITY, REHOSPITALIZATION, AND MORTALITY: THE MEDICAL FATE OF PATIENTS AFTER DISCHARGE FROM THE HOSPITAL

INTRODUCTION

This chapter focuses on a key aspect of "outcome" for the men in the study population over the course of the year: their physical health level. Here we report on data on the proportions who died and survived, as well as information on rehospitalizations, reported symptoms, and the absence of illness.

In addition to the reporting of morbidity and mortality, we review the results of a series of exploratory efforts to determine variables associated with death or illness pattern during the period after hospitalization (see, for examples, Beard et al., 1960; Schiffman, 1970; Kannel and Feinleib, 1972; Rosenman et al., 1970; Shapiro et al., 1965, 1970; Weinblatt et al., 1968; Theorell and Rahe, 1975).[1] These variables include (a) a series of social identity items, (b) behavioral and attitudinal materials as indicated by patients in interviews, and

(c) assessments and predictions made through question-naires by the physicians providing care for the patients. These materials were explored in an effort to answer the question, "What variables in the background of the patient and his characteristics early in the illness appear to be associated with prospects of survival, rehospitalization, and recurrence of illness during the study year?"[2]

METHODS AND SOURCES
FOR CLASSIFICATION

Although the nature of the study population and the methods of this study are presented in Chapter 1 and are given in greater detail in the Appendix, some recapitulation seems desirable as we discuss the data. Readers interested in a more detailed review of the procedures employed in relation to this chapter will find further information in the Notes section at the end.

The study population, it will be recalled, consisted of men who fit the strict medical criteria for eligibility and who were about to leave the hospital after treatment for a first myocardial infarction. They were also men whose course of illness in the hospital was characterized medically as "without complications." We are dealing therefore with a select group, one which is not representative of the total admissions for myocardial infarctions in the participating hospitals.

Further, the period of risk which we report upon extends from the T_1 interview, at approximately three weeks post-infarct, to the T_3 interview, one year after admission. The period is therefore slightly less than a year, and it excludes the period of maximum mortality in heart disease—the first few days after the acute onset of the attack. The study population was chosen on the basis of criteria designed to permit the investigation of differential response to crisis over an extended period. To understand it in these terms aids in drawing appropriate conclusions about morbidity and mortality in a select population.

The materials for this report on mortality and morbidity were derived from two principal sources: (a) the interview at T_3 with the patients and (b) medical questionnaires completed by their physicians at the time of the T_2 and T_3 interviews with the patients. In addition to reporting on subsequent rehospitalizations, the physicians were asked to provide information regarding development of disorders associated with arteriosclerotic heart disease (ASHD) and other significant disease processes in the patients during the study year.[3]

The size of the study population with which we are concerned in this chapter deserves special note. In tracing the illness experience of the patients over the year, we begin our report with a total of 348 men. This group consists of all those who fit criteria for the study, who were interviewed at T_1, and who left the hospital. Three of the men died before the T_2 interview. As they met initial criteria, we have included them insofar as their health history is clearly relevant to the aims of this chapter. However, since they could not take part in the T_2 interview, they are necessarily excluded from the analysis which deals with that phase. Accordingly, we focus upon the surviving 345 patients in subsequent chapters of this volume.

DEATHS AND REHOSPITALIZATIONS: THE QUESTION OF HEALTH LEVEL

Deaths and Readmissions to Hospital

In terms of health level over the course of the study year, the patients can be differentiated into three groups: (a) those who died, (b) those who were rehospitalized and survived, and (c) those who were not rehospitalized after the discharge for their myocardial infarction. These three categories thus indicate relatively clear-cut groups in terms of illness level: (a) those who were so seriously ill that they died; (b) those who came to the attention of physicians and were considered sufficiently ill to require hospitalization, and who survived the full year; and finally, (c) those who lived the full study year and were not adjudged by a physician to require rehospitalization for illness

These groups are not perfectly exclusive, of course. Some who were not rehospitalized may have had ailments which some physicians might commit to care; those who were actually rehospitalized may not have been as ill as some who were not rehospitalized. For working purposes, however, these three categories designate three types of illness experience ranked, at least crudely, by severity.

The third category, the non-rehospitalized, can be further subdivided by illness level, based on physician reports. Thus, one group may be characterized as (1) not rehospitalized but reported by the physician as having developed disorders associated with ASHD or other significant disease processes and as (2) not rehospitalized and not reported by physicians as being in category (1). This differentiation is, of course, not as clear-cut and unequivocal as the categories based on the information as to whether a patient died or was rehospitalized, but it does provide a further useful perspective on subsequent illness experience after T_1.

In Table 1 we present data on the mortality, hospitalization, and reported illness experience of the patient population at the time of T_3. The percentage information is offered, for purposes of completeness, on two groups. In Column 1 the percentages are based on the total study population of 348 men, including some

who did not participate at T_3 but whom we know survived (N=39). As we do not have further information on
their rehospitalization and health history, the 39 men
stand as a separate category of survivors. In the third
column of the table, however, these men are excluded
from percentages, in order that we may examine the
data on all those men for whom we have adequate and
comparable information. These percentages are therefore based on a total of 309 men, i.e., all participants at
T_3 plus those who did not survive the year.[4]

As may be seen in Table 1, of an initial patient
population of 348, 16 men died during the course of the
study year (T_1 to T_3). Almost all of these were deceased
for heart-related reasons.[5] Thirteen suffered an acute
myocardial infarction, and one died of heart disease
other than myocardial infarction. One patient died by
accidental means. The cause of death of the sixteenth
man is not known, since he moved to a distant state
before his demise. At the time of admission for the first
heart attack, however, he was diagnosed as also having
cancer, and he was subsequently rehospitalized for this
condition at least three times over the months before his
death.

As the table shows, 46 men were rehospitalized
during the course of the year either for heart disease
alone, or for heart-related problems in addition to other
illnesses. An additional 19 men were rehospitalized for
treatment of non-heart ailments. Among the men who
were rehospitalized for heart-related ailments, such
diagnoses were given as coronary insufficiency, problems
with anti-coagulant medication and recurrence of
myocardial infarction. This latter group, i.e., hospitalized
for myocardial infarction, consisted of 14 men. Diagnoses for those rehospitalized for non-heart ailments
included pneumonia, asthmatic bronchitis, diverticulitis,
hemoptysis of unknown etiology, kidney stone, lung

Table 1. Medical Fate During Study Year. From T_1 to T_3.

Medical Fate	N	Medical Fate at One Year (T_3) Percent of T_1 Study Cohort N = 348	Medical Fate at One Year (T_3) Percent of T_3 Study Cohort (Excluding Case Losses) N = 309
Deceased			
Heart Disease:	14	4.0	4.5
Non-heart Causes:	2	.6	.6
Rehospitalized With Survival			
Heart Disease:	46	13.2	14.9
Non-heart Causes:	19	5.5	6.2
Not Rehospitalized			
With ASHD Associated Disorders and/or Other Disease Processes:*	81	23.3	26.2
No Additional Disorders:**	116	33.3	37.6
No Data on Health Level From M.D.:***	31	8.9	10.0
Survived - No Further Information:****	39	11.2	Excluded
Total	348	100.0	100.0

* Patients in this category were described by their physicians in questionnaires at T_3 as having developed (a) disorders associated with arteriosclerotic heart disease during year and/or (b) other significant disease processes.

** Patients in this category were not rehospitalized, nor were they classified by their physicians as having developed disorders or disease processes as in previous category.

*** No questionnaires regarding these patients were returned by their physicians at T_3, and classification by presence or absence of medically reported disease is not possible.

**** This group consists of patients who withdrew from the study or were otherwise inaccessible for the T_3 interview.

abscess, injuries from car accidents, and surgery for problems including appendicitis, hernias, rectal cancer, hemorrhoids, disc, gall bladder disease and ulcers.

Most of those shown in the table as rehospitalized went back into the hospital only a single additional time during the study year. In the case of the heart disease group, however, a relatively large proportion (40 percent) had two hospitalizatons or more. Thus, of the 46 surviving rehospitalized men, 28 went back into the hospital once for "heart disease" reasons, 15 were rehospitalized with heart disease two or more times subsequent to their first experience, and the remaining three had two or more subsequent rehospitalizations, at least one of which was for heart disease.

Among those 19 patients who were rehospitalized for treatment of non-heart illnesses or conditions, 15 had one rehospitalization and four had two or more stays in the hospital.

As Table 1 also shows, 81 mén, while not rehospitalized, were described by their physicians as having developed disorders associated with ASHD and/or other significant disease processes during the study year.[6] It is likely that this number is an underestimation, since a segment of those physicians who did not respond might have included some of their patients in this group.[7] The disorders associated with ASHD included diabetes, arrhythmias, anginal syndrome, coronary insufficiency, congestive heart failure, hypertension and complications of drug therapy. In a few cases, patients were reported as having other significant disease processes, including severe anxiety with depression, cholelethiasis, adhesive capsulitis of the shoulder, and ulcer symptoms.

In summary, it is most useful here to use Column 3 in Table 1 for reference, insofar as the base consists of those patients on whom we have the more ample data. There, as we see, subsequent to their hospital discharge more than half the study population suffered further serious disease problems during the study year. Five percent died, and approximately 20 percent more were rehospitalized one or more more times and survived. The remainder, while not rehospitalized, developed other significant illness, as reported by their physicians. In the majority of cases, these deaths, rehospitalizations and illnesses were heart-disease related.

Once again, we must emphasize, caution must be used in interpreting these statistics. This population, as we have noted, was a relatively elite group from the standpoint of previous health history. It seems probable that the picture of death, rehospitalization and additional illness during the study year would have been even more grave, if, for example, it had included men who had been treated for illnesses previous to their first hospitalization, men whose cases were classified as "complicated," and patients over 60 years old.

MORTALITY, MORBIDITY, AND ASSOCIATED VARIABLES

After considering the differences in the medical fates of the patients at one year after their myocardial infarction, we next explored whether particular demographic, social, and psychological variables present at T_1 and T_2 were associated with such fates. We were also interested in determining whether these variables might have predictive value for similar study populations.

In line with these concerns, we examined a series of variables in relation to the medical outcome measures. These procedures and cross-tabulations were reviewed in Chapter 1. The specific items for examination were selected on the basis of their relevance to a series of theoretical assumptions and beliefs concerning the relationship of demographic, social and psychological factors to the etiology and course of illness (Jenkins, 1971). The variables included such items as social status characteristics, age, marital status, religion, ethnic origin, measures of work stress before the illness, cigarette smoking, pattern of reported physical symptoms, level of physical activity before the illness, as well as indices of marital disagreement, and personality self-rating items.[8]

In such a screening operation a percentage of apparently significant relationships will occur purely by chance. Despite this possibility, the exploratory effort to determine correlates of medical fate yielded few relationships worthy of note. We found only a minimal number of social and psychological variables which were in the direction of meaningful relationships with medical variables.

Findings on at least two particular sets of data deserve review in terms of their relationship to medical outcome. These are (a) social status characteristics of the patients and (b) physician predictions about the physical status of the patients at one year.

Social Status and Occupational Type

In recent years a substantial body of literature has appeared in which evidence is set forth concerning the role of social-status factors in the etiology and epidemiology of heart disease, mental disease, psychosomatic disorders, and a variety of other ailments. In heart disease, as well as in other areas, the controversy remains unresolved in regard to the association of social status with the onset and course of the illness (see, for example, Antonovsky, 1967, 1968; Dohrenwend and Dohrenwend, 1969; Graham and Reeder, 1972; Kadushin, 1967; Langner and Michael, 1963; Leighton, 1959; Levine and Scotch, 1970; Mechanic, 1968;

Shekelle et al., 1969; Syme et al., 1964).

In view of the earnest and unsettled controversy as to the role of social status factors in heart disease, several measures of social status were included for the exploratory cross-tabulations with medical fate. In Table 2 these appear in relation to death or rehospitalization of patients for heart-related reasons during the course of the study year.

Is health level, as reflected by rehospitalization or by death from heart disease during the year, related to social status variables? In Table 2, on superficial inspection, a relationship appears to be evident. Closer examination refutes this, however, and the statistical tests give a clear negative picture as well. For example, on the education variable, the difference in percentage rehospitalized between the two extreme groups ("college" versus "three years high school or less") is only 14 percent.

On the occupational variable there seems at first to be a more striking association, as the difference between the extreme categories ("executive-professionals" versus "semi-skilled and unskilled") is more substantial—about 25 percent. When we examine all four categories in relation to each other, however, the differences seem less impressive. The difference between "small business, white collar" and the "semi-skilled, unskilled" is only 12 percent. The difference in proportion between "small business" and "skilled" is less than one percent. Similar small percentage differences appear in the third segment of the table dealing with the percent rehospitalized and the array of patients by family income. The superficial appearance of relationship may also be affected in part by the small numbers in cells. When cells are combined to increase the number for analysis, the initial appearance of relationships clearly does not hold.

Table 2. Medical Outcome During Study Year. Percent Deceased Patients and Rehospitalized Survivors. Heart Disease Patients Only. T_1 to T_3. By Social Status Indicators.

	Deceased or Rehospitalized On Account of Heart Disease (Percent)		Survivors Not Rehospitalized (Percent)		Total Study Group*
Educational Level					
One Year of College or More	10.8	(8)	89.2	(66)	74
High School Graduate	21.8	(20)	78.2	(72)	92
Three Years High School or Less	24.6	(29)	75.4	(89)	118
Total		(57)		(227)	284
Chi-square = 5.60, d.f. = 2, p<.10, gamma = .26					
Occupational Category					
High Level Executives or Professionals	8.8	(5)	91.2	(52)	57
Small Business, White Collar	21.2	(21)	78.8	(78)	99
Skilled	22.0	(11)	78.0	(39)	50
Semiskilled and Unskilled	25.3	(20)	74.7	(59)	79
Total		(57)		(228)	285
Chi-square = 6.10, d.f. = 3, p<.20; gamma = .24					
Total Family Income in Year Before the Illness					
$15,000 or More	12.9	(4)	87.1	(27)	31
$12,500 - $14,999	16.0	(4)	84.0	(21)	25
$10,000 - $12,499	16.0	(8)	84.0	(42)	50
$ 7,500 - $ 9,999	20.4	(19)	79.6	(74)	93
Less Than $ 7,500	26.5	(22)	73.5	(61)	83
Total		(57)		(225)	282
Chi-square = 3.90, d.f. = 4, p<.50; gamma = .21					

* Differences in totals are due to differences in availability of information concerning education, occupation and income. Thirty-nine men are omitted who survived the study year, but for whom we have no information on illness patterns.

that at least some suggestive weak trends are present in all three measures. Certainly the matter deserves more substantial inquiry by other investigators with access to larger study populations.[9]

Physician Prediction as an Index of Optimism and Outcome at One Year

A second type of variable associated with medical fate of the patient consisted of the prognostic ratings made by their physicians. At the time of T_2, physicians were requested to complete a questionnaire which included a prediction as to the activity level of the patient at one year after the myocardial infarction. The physician was requested to classify the patient as of one year according to one of the following categories:

1. will return to full activity without significant impairment,
2. will return to full activity but with significant modifications in daily living schedule and activities,
3. will have definite residual limitations on his work and activities.

The categories are based upon those of the New York Heart Association and are well known to most physicians treating heart patients in the geographic area of the study (Criteria Committee, New York Heart Association, 1964).

Classification of patients into these categories is based on a number of factors, including the actual condition of the patient, the degree of knowledge of the patient by the physician, the clinical judgment and sophistication of the physician, and his willingness to state a categorical prognosis. Making this kind of predictive rating is consistent with the training and clinical practice of physicians (Peel et al., 1972). In order to treat patients, the physician must necessarily make some assessment of the current condition, total situation, and long-term prognosis. Upon such judgments as these, the physician designs the therapeutic program and advises the patient.

Given the fact that physicians, as part of the task of medical practice, must make judgments about each case and its course, we attempted to determine the relationships between one type of physician judgment and subsequent medical history of the heart patients. Thus, the prognostic ratings are operationally defined here as expressions of optimism-pessimism concerning the course of the illness.

At the extreme end of the "optimism-pessimism scale," we assume that physician to be optimistic who indicates that his patient at one year will be engaged in full activity without significant impairment. We assume that physician to be pessimistic if he foresaw the patient at one year as having "definite residual limitations on his work and activities." Category 2 may be seen as intermediate on the "optimism-pessimism scale."

The physicians, it must be emphasized, were not asked to predict death or rehospitalization during the year. We are using their rating reflecting optimism-pessimism as one of the "antecedent variables" describing patients at T_2, in addition to the many other social and psychological indicators.

When the total number of physician ratings at T_2 are examined, it is apparent that most show optimism concerning the condition of their patients at one year after their hospital admission. Of the 324 patients for whom ratings are available, 60 percent were rated in Category 1 (most optimistic) and 28 percent were in Category 2. Only 11 percent were placed in Category 3 (most pessimistic). For the remaining one percent (comprising four men), their physicians gave no prognostic rating, indicating either "insufficient information" or "don't know."

Table 3.   Medical Predictions at T_2 on Patients at T_3.   By Medical Fate of Patients.   Deaths and Rehospitalization During Period T_2 to T_3.

Medical Predictions	Dead or Rehospitalized		Not Rehospitalized	Total Percent	Total N
	Heart Disease	Non-heart Illness			
1. Optimism - "without impairment"	14.7 (25)	5.8 (10)	79.5 (136)	100.0	171
2. "Significant modifications"	16.7 (14)	10.7 (9)	72.6 (61)	100.0	84
3. Pessimism - "residual limitations"	50.0 (15)	3.3 (1)	46.7 (14)	100.0	30

Chi-square - 23.49, d.f. - 4, p<.001 for total population.
Chi-square = 20.03, d.f. = 2, p<.001 non-heart illness excluded.

Considering the patients at the end of the year when their medical fate had become apparent, what had their physicians predicted about them earlier in terms of our optimism-pessimism criterion? As Table 3 shows, there is an apparent relationship between physician prediction rating and the outcome, if we look at the percentage of men dead or rehospitalized in terms of each individual prognostic category. Thus, of 171 men who received rating #1, only 15 percent were dead or rehospitalized for heart-related causes during the study year. Of those who received the most pessimistic physician rating at T_2, however, 50 percent had been rehospitalized or were dead for heart-related causes.

These data can also be examined through reference to physician reports on illness level during the year, as well as hospitalization and mortality. For this purpose we compared three groups: (1) Dead or rehospitalized: heart disease (N=54), (2) Not rehospitalized but reported as having significant additional ASHD disorders and/or disease (N=77), and (3) Not rehospitalized and not reported as having additional disorders or disease (N=113). These categories thus reflect three levels of reported illness, with (1) representing the most severe and (3) representing the least severe.[10] When seen in this way, in relation to physician optimism-pessimism rating, the data are not markedly different from those reported in Table 3. In brief, consideration of the additional aspect of severity of illness during the year did not make a difference in the results.

While the data on rehospitalization and illness level may be subject to varying interpretations because of the system of classification, it is possible to classify patients by a simple and unequivocal method: whether they died or survived the year. Of the 14 men who died of heart disease, 10 had received ratings in the questionnaires by their physicians at T_2. The numbers are too small to permit generalization from the data, but they give a picture consistent with that evident when the larger population is considered. Of the 10 men, four had been rated in the most optimistic category. Two men were rated in Category 2, and three were given the most pessimistic rating, Category 3. When these men are considered in relation to the total numbers in each of the three optimism-pessimism categories, they constitute the following proportions: three percent of the total number in Category 1, two percent of the number in Category 2, and ten percent of those in Category 3.

In summary, of the many variables examined in terms of their possible relationships to the patient's health level during the study year subsequent to his first hospital discharge, the physician optimism pessimism index proved most productive. Although the physicians were not asked specifically to predict death or rehospitalization, it seems that their rating on future activity level or functional capacity of the patient had some statistical relationship to these "death-rehospitalization" outcomes.

SUMMARY

This chapter has reviewed aspects of the medical fate of the men comprising the specially screened and selected study population of this research. This group of heart patients had been discharged from the hospital and met criteria for age, previous health status, and "non-complicated" hospital course. Approximately 95 percent survived to one year after their first infarction. The group exhibited a mixed health picture, however, as portrayed by the application of differing analytic criteria. For example, while only 5 percent of the total population died, about 20 percent were rehospitalized, most for heart-related causes.

According to reports from physicians, approximately one-fourth of the patients, aside from those who were rehospitalized and deceased, were described as having developed disorders during the year associated with ASHD and/or other significant disease processes.

It can be pointed out that at the end of the study year half the patient group had remained relatively free of further serious illness. For the remainder, however, the period after their initial hospitalization was one of further hospital admissions and/or other evidence of serious health problems.

Explorations were made to isolate demographic,

social, and psychological variables which might be predictive of "medical fate," i.e., death, rehospitalizaton or serious illness. No significant associations were found. Predictions by the physicians of the patients, when employed as measures of optimism or pessimism, appeared of some value, however, as a means of assessing "medical fate" for the study year.

NOTES

1. Detailed comparisons between the results of these studies as well as our own can be made only with caution, since they differ in terms of such factors as criteria for selection of study populations, research methods, and other aspects of study design.
2. As noted in a footnote in Chapter 1, several key symbols will be used as designations of the three principal time stages of this study. "T_1" refers to the period in the hospital, approximately three weeks after admission for the first myocardial infarction. "T_2" refers to the period at one month after discharge from the hospital, approximately seven weeks after the admission to the hospital. "T_3" refers to the period one year after the initial hospital admission. It thus designates also the end of the study year. As interviews with the patients were held at the time of T_1, T_2 and T_3, these symbols are also used in the text to refer to the interviews themselves as well as the time period when they occurred.
3. The specific questions addressed to physicians were:
    1. "During the past year, has the patient developed any of these disorders associated with Arteriosclerotic Heart Disease?" A checklist consisted of the following items: "Another myocardial infarction, coronary insufficiency, anginal syndrome, congestive heart failure, arrythmia, diabetes, hypertension, complication of drug therapy."

2. "Have any other significant disease processes arisen in the past year?" If the answer was "yes," the physician was asked to specify.

Employing this method, initial definition of "significant disease process" depends upon the clinical judgment of the physician, an effort consistent with the usual requirements of clinical practice. The diseases reported were then reviewed by the Medical Director of the project, ascertaining whether the items reported were indeed "significant disease processes," as they would be identified by experienced clinicians employing standards of common practice in medicine. Specific examples of the items reported by physicians in response to the question appear in the next section of this chapter.

4. Data accounting for all patients at each stage appear in Appendix A.

5. *Evidence of Myocardial Infarction Subsequent to the Initial Admission.* Since the project as a whole is concerned with factors in differential response to the crisis of a heart attack, one of the crucial concerns was the recurrence of the illness. In the case of patients who died, information of myocardial infarction as a cause of death was obtained from their physicians, from hospitals, or from the State Bureau of Vital Statistics. In the case of patients surviving the year, data were obtained first through the report of the physicians in response to the questionnaires compiled at one year. In addition, information drawn from the T_3 interview with the patient was employed. In cases where the patient reported that he had an additional myocardial infarction, but where the physician reported none, investigation was carried out to resolve the discrepancy. In these instances, the report by the physician prevailed. In 31 cases where there was no questionnaire from the physician, the appropriate hospitals were consulted as needed to check on accuracy of patient reports concerning admission and diagnosis.

The data on subsequent myocardial infarction, it must be stressed, come from these various physician, record, and patient sources. We have no information on the silent infarct, or the non-reported symptoms which were actually myocardial infarction. It was not within the resources or scope of this research to carry out the intensive physical examinations of patients which would be required to document clinical course over the year.

6. See Reference 3 above for explanation.

7. We are dealing here simply with physician report on presence or absence of patient illness. It enables us in at least a rough way to

distinguish between two groups of patients: (1) those who came to medical attention for additional ailments during the course of the year and (2) those who did not.

The absence of reported illness does not, of course, mean that patients in Group 2 were "well." Indeed, the fact that some may have had ailments which they did not bring to medical attention serves as a confounding factor in statistical analysis comparing Groups 1 and 2. Since some of the patients in Group 2 really belonged in Group 1, this would serve to reduce any distinctions between the two groups found in our analysis. This factor must therefore be kept in mind in the evaluation of data comparing the two groups. The finding of lack of significant differences on a variable may be influenced by this factor. Further, when a significant difference is found, the level of significance may be reduced by this factor as well.

8. As the variables are part of the core analysis for this book and are discussed in the various succeeding chapters of this volume, we will not list and describe each of them here. As the text indicates, the screening effort produced mainly a negative result.

9. We feel impelled, however, to report at this point that approximately eight years after the infarction, the influence of social class is clearly evident. For example, in our most recent study, conducted as a follow-up to the work we report here, preliminary data show that among the sub-cohort of men who were rehospitalized for a second or third infarction, the incidence of death among semiskilled and unskilled patients was considerably higher than it was for all other occupational levels. More specifically, 66 percent of these men in the lowest occupational group had died versus 38 percent for all other occupational categories. These data will be reported in detail in subsequent publications.

10. The total number (N=244) differs from the totals appearing in Table 3 reporting on physician ratings on optimism-pessimism. (N=285). These data in the text exclude patients who were dead, rehospitalized or ill because of diseases or conditions other than heart disease. The summary data in the table include all patients on whom physician ratings were given.

Chapter 3

EMPLOYMENT AND WORK EXPERIENCE AFTER HOSPITALIZATION

INTRODUCTION

Work is one of the key elements in the "armory of resources" of heart disease patients that influences the course and outcome of recovery and rehabilitation. Aside from providing means of economic support, it performs a variety of other functions, affecting mental and physical health, personal identity, self-esteem, social well-being, family relations and *Weltanschauung* (Caplan et al., 1975; Copp, 1965 and 1966; Safilios-Rothschild, 1970; Whyte, 1961). What is the experience of the patient population in regard to this key area? In answering this question, we will examine some of the ways in which work as a resource operates for differing subsegments of the patient population group.

In the literature centering specifically on rehabilitation of heart patients, a primary focus is often given to the area of work. The extent to which patients are able to return to their former occupations, their capacity to engage in full-time employment, and the length of the period of disability before work return have all served as important indicators of progress in rehabilitation and recovery (see, for example, Biorck, 1964; Crain and Missal, 1956; Croog et al., 1968; Garrity, 1973; Pell and D'Alonzo, 1964; Shapiro et al., 1972; Sharland, 1964). It is to this area which we now turn, considering both the objective data on pattern of return as well as a series of materials on the subjective meaning of work for the patients.

The first section of the chapter reports on work plans, prospects, and concerns in the early stages after the heart attack. The second section reviews the experience of the patients in regard to work over the course of the year following the heart attack. Main areas discussed are patterns of return to work, changes in the nature of the work, and the problems patients reported during the year. The third section covers (a) changes in the perception of the role of work in the etiology of the illness, (b) perceptions of the nature of stresses in the employment situation, and (c) various adaptive responses to these. A fourth section considers briefly some issues concerning health level and its relationship to the employment experience. Finally, we recapitulate some of the materials in the chapter dealing with ways in which work operates as a resource in recovery and rehabilitation.

For purposes of this chapter, the main analytic variable is that of occupational status. In preliminary analysis it was immediately apparent that the work fate, problems, and concerns of patients were linked in important ways to where those patients were located on the occupational scale. Occupation, in fact, provided a consistently more useful means of differentiating patients than did health level or other items.

The four-category occupational classification is

employed throughout the chapter.[1] Thus, Group 1 refers to professionals and higher level executives, Group 2 to small businessmen and white collar workers, Group 3 to skilled workers, and Group 4 to semiskilled and unskilled laborers. Since the experience of the semiskilled and unskilled laborers is distinctive from that of other categories, they are kept as a separate group.

THE EARLY PERIOD: WORK EXPERIENCE AND JOB PLANS

Job Plans During Hospital Stay and Recuperation at Home

While the patients were still in the hospital, data were obtained at the T_1 interview in regard to their work plans.[2] At a time shortly before their discharge, most patients had already made decisions about their work. Most (81.5 percent) indicated that they planned to return to the same job they held before they became ill.[3] Only 11 percent reported uncertainty about the matter.

Within the group of men who planned to return to the same job, most planned also to continue the same type of work they had pursued before becoming ill (82 percent).[4] A few (five percent) indicated uncertainty about whether they would change their type of work, and 13 percent reported that they would not do the same type of work when they returned to their job. Thus, looking at the population as a whole, it would appear that most assumed an optimistic outlook, with the majority planning to return to their previous employment and to perform the same type of work.

Significant differences in job plans appear when men from differing occupational groups are compared. As may be seen in Table 1, a greater proportion of

Table 1. Job Intentions at T_1 and T_2. By Percent Within Occupational Group.

	Percent of Cohort "Yes" Response	Percent Giving "Yes" Response Occupational Group				"p"*
		I	II	III	IV	
At T_1						
Expect to return to same job as before illness?	81.5 (278)(341)	95.2 (60)(63)	91.5 (108)(118)	79.0 (49)(62)	62.2 (61)(98)	p<.001
Expect to do same type of work as before at same job?	82.0 (228)(278)	91.7 (55)(60)	81.5 (88)(108)	81.6 (40)(49)	73.8 (45)(61)	p<.10
At T_2**						
Expect to return to same job as before illness?	69.2 (180)(260)	82.1 (32)(39)	83.7 (72)(86)	65.1 (28)(43)	52.2 (48)(92)	p<.001

* "p": significance level as indicated by Chi-square test.

** Computations based solely upon patients who were not yet back at work at T_2.

executive and white collar worker categories indicate that they plan to return to the same job. Among those returning, moreover, higher proportions of the executives and professionals planned to carry on with the same type of work. Thus, at T_1 it would appear that in regard to making a decision about returning to work and to carrying out the same type of work, it was the blue collar workers who in highest proportions were considering changes.

By the time of the second interview, at approximately one month after discharge from hospital, a substantial proportion of the patients had already returned to work on either a part-time or full-time basis. Of the 261 men who had not returned to work when the T_2 interview took place, however, essentially the same decision pattern regarding change in location of employment was evident. Among these, 69 percent indicated that they planned to return to the same job. Further, the pattern of intention to return varied among men of the different occupational categories, as shown in Table 1. Once again the groups showed significant statistical differences in their responses.[5]

At the time of the second interview, as Table 1 shows, the proportion of men in each of the four occupational categories who planned to return to the same place dropped somewhat below the earlier proportions. This is due to the fact that many men who at T_1 had planned to return to the same job had already done so by T_2. With their removal, it should be noted that the situation of Groups 3 and 4 contrasts more sharply with that of Groups 1 and 2. In fact, within Group 4 in particular, approximately *half* of those still out of work at Stage 2 anticipated a job change.

Plans for Changes

In addition to the larger issues of change in job and type of work, patients were asked questions at T_2 about changes in plans which the illness had necessitated. One month after discharge from hospital, 30 percent responded in the affirmative to the question, "Have you had to make changes in plans in regard to your work or your job?" The greater proportion of negative responses to this query is consistent with other responses reflecting general optimism or possible denial expressed by the majority of patients. Nevertheless, a sizeable proportion responded in the affirmative, indicating alteration of a major segment of their lives. It is useful to examine the nature of these responses in detail.

Table 2. Ranking by Magnitude: Changes in Job Plans Among Those Specifying Changes at T_2.
N = 103*

Area Specified	Percent
Do Lighter Work, Same Setting	36.9 (38)
Reduce Hours	28.2 (29)
Do Lighter Work, Different Job	23.3 (24)
Reduce Responsibility	12.6 (13)
Stop Second Job	2.9 (3)
Give Up Previously Planned Occupational Changes	1.0 (1)
Total	108

* Percentages are based on individual items in relation to number of persons reporting change, and they are not cumulative. It should be specifically noted that while the total number of men equals 103, the number of changes they reported equals 108.

Looking at the 30 percent of the study population who reported alterations in plans, some general themes emerge. In Table 2 the reported changes are ranked by magnitude, and they are presented as a percentage of the total number of men who reported changes (N=103). In the main, the tenor of these changes is in the direction of reducing activities and responsibilities. The question was an open-ended one and elicited concerns which were salient. It is worth noting, however, that at this point not a single man mentioned the possibility of retiring. Further, though a relatively large proportion of the *total* study group held more than one job in the period before the heart attack (18 percent), only three men indicated that they planned to give up their second job. On the whole, most of the 103 men (95 percent) mentioned only one change which they anticipated, while virtually all the remainder specified two.

Predictions and Concerns

At the time of the T$_2$ interview, many patients appeared to have relatively optimistic views in regard to the potential impact of the disease upon their work lives and their employment careers. Table 3 indicates some of their areas of concern. Patients were first asked a general question, "After an illness a person may go back to a job and find nothing has changed. In other cases he can expect problems and changes. What effect do you think your illness will have on the nature of the work that you do?" Among those patients who responded to this query, about half simply answered "None" (54 percent). A sizeable number, however, did envision some negative effects of the illness upon their work.

All patients were then asked a series of questions concerning effects on particular aspects of work. Nearly one-fourth of the men foresaw an influence of the illness upon their salary and earnings. Here, surprisingly, there were no significant variations by occupational type.

Table 3. Reported Perceptions of Future Effects of Heart Attack on Aspects of Work. By Percent Within Occupational Groups. At T_2 *

	Percent of Cohort "Yes" Response	Percent Giving "Yes" Response Occupational Group				"p"**
		I	II	III	IV	
Illness will have some effects on nature of work performed.	46.3 (132)(285)	37.5 (21)(56)	39.4 (41)(104)	50.0 (22)(44)	59.3 (48)(81)	p<.02
Effects on salary or earnings.	23.3 (68)(292)	26.9 (14)(52)	20.0 (22)(110)	19.2 (10)(52)	28.2 (22)(78)	NS
Effects on promotion or long-term advancement.	20.1 (55)(273)	11.1 (5)(45)	18.6 (18)(97)	20.8 (10)(48)	26.5 (22)(83)	NS
Raise problems with employer or fellow workers.	15.3 (48)(294)	12.0 (6)(50)	10.0 (10)(100)	17.6 (9)(51)	24.7 (23)(93)	p<.05

* "Don't Know" and "No Response" categories have been excluded. Because of the difference in the numbers of patients answering each question, the "N's" are reported in parentheses underneath the percentages.

** "p": significance level as indicated by Chi-square test. NS = not significant.

About one-fifth perceived some possible effects on their opportunities for promotion or long-term advancement. Finally, 16 percent of the total considered that the illness might raise possible problems with their employers or fellow workers. As Table 3 shows, these problems were anticipated by higher proportions of semiskilled and unskilled workers than by professionals and executives.[6]

The data in the table are based upon the total population at T_2. The situation of the self-employed professional and the individual entrepreneur may be considered to be different from that of the employed worker, since he has greater control over his work activities, he is relieved of concerns about an employer, and the prospects for his promotion may not be at issue. The same data were reexamined, therefore, to include only those who were salaried employees. The pattern of relationships shown in Table 3 was not changed by this procedure.

In their predictions about the future impact on work, the patients on the whole showed relative optimism and security when the T_2 interviews were carried out. The greatest negative impact was foreseen by blue-collar workers. In response to individual questions in particular, at least one out of four of the semiskilled and unskilled workers foresaw problems in income, advancement, and interpersonal relations as consequences of the disease.

T_3: ONE YEAR AFTER THE HEART ATTACK

Work Situation and Employment History

At one year after the heart attack, when patients were interviewed again, they were asked about their work experience of the previous year and the ways in which their expectations had materialized. Among those patients who participated in interviews at the third stage, there were several notable features in regard to their employment status at the time. As may be seen in Table 4, most of the respondents (84 percent) were employed either full-time or part-time when seen again. Of the 16.5 percent who were currently unemployed, most of these (12 percent) had not worked at all during the year, while the remainder were out of work at the time of T_3.

Table 4. Employment Status at T_3.
Percent by Occupational Group. Total T_3 Cohort.

	Percent Cohort	Percent Occupational Group			
		I	II	III	IV
Employment Status					
A. Currently Full-time	76.4	91.4	80.4	74.1	62.7
B. Currently Part-time	7.2	3.4	10.3	9.3	4.8
C. Currently Unemployed*	4.5	3.4	3.1	5.6	6.0
D. Unemployed Throughout Year	12.0	1.7	6.2	11.1	26.5
Total Unemployed (C + D)	16.5	5.1	9.3	16.7	32.5
Total N	292	58	97	54	83

* Category 'C' includes men who were currently unemployed at T_3 and had earlier been employed at some time during the year.

It seems apparent from Table 4 that the occupational status of the men is linked vitally with their employment experience during the year. While only one man from the executive-professional category remained out of work, as many as one-fourth of the semiskilled and unskilled did not work at all (26.5 percent). Moreover, the prospects for full-time employment were apparently best for those in the higher occupational categories. As seen in the first row, there is a linear association of full-time employment status with occupational category, and the proportion of executive-professionals who were full-time exceeds that of the semiskilled and unskilled by nearly 30 percent. The explanation for this finding, it must be emphasized, does not appear to come from the pattern of illness or the recurrence. As was shown in Chapter 2, there was no clear relationship between status and rehospitalization during the year, nor was there a relationship of status with severity of the illness (as classified according to the various physician and patient assessments).[7]

Perhaps a more dramatic aspect of the work situation is the report on current employment status, as seen among the various occupational groups. At the time of T_3, fully one-third of the men in Group 4 were unemployed. This proportion stands in sharp contrast to that of men in other occupational categories, particularly as compared with Group 1, which had only 5 percent unemployed.

What were the reasons why one segment of the total population remained out of work over the course of the entire year? Figure 1 summarizes the patients' responses.

Figure 1
Reported Reasons for Remaining Unemployed Throughout Study Year

Number	Explanation by Patient
11	Physician advised patient to retire
10	Patient did not feel well enough to work
4	Physician advised patient to look for another job, and he has not yet found one
4	Physician advised patient to "take it easy"
4	Patient unable to find suitable type of work
2	Employer unwilling to hire or rehire patient

As Figure 1 shows, primary reported explanations for unemployment were based on advice from a physician. The feelings of the patients and their views of the illness were also prominent, with patients reporting that they did not feel well enough to work or that the physician advised them "to take it easy." Some patients reported that they were unable to find suitable employment, and two pointed out directly that they were out of work because of refusals of employers to hire them. In sum, nearly half the unemployed (19 out of 35 men) referred to some aspect of physician advice, with the remainder referring to their own subjective state or their problems in finding work appropriate to their health condition.[8]

Yet, though these men had been unemployed for a year, nearly half of them indicated that they eventually planned to return to work. Nearly all of these had no intention of returning to the same type of employment as before, however. Thus at one year after the T_1 hospital admission those unemployed were most agreed on one thing: that they would not do the same type of work they had performed prior to their illness.

Work Return: Pattern

Of those patients who returned to work, over half had gone back within 90 days following their discharge from the hospital. Nearly 30 percent had returned before 60 days had elapsed.

Interval between Work Return and Date of Discharge
Among those returning to work in 11 months after discharge

Less than two months	27.5 percent
Two months, less than three	27.8
Three months, less than four	18.7
Four months, less than six	13.0
Six months to 11	13.0

The proportions of men from different occupational

groups did not differ in terms of date of work return, except for those who did not return for four months or more. Here, there was a negative association between occupational status and relative slowness in returning to work. Of all employed patients in each occupational category who returned to work after the lapse of four or more months following discharge from hospital, the breakdown was: Group 1—17.5 percent, Group 2—20 percent, Group 3—25 percent, and Group 4—43 percent.

These figures on work return take on additional meaning when related to data on men unemployed throughout the year. Estimating that discharge from hospital occurred three weeks postadmission, on the average, it is possible to calculate the proportion of men in each occupational group who were in an unemployed status nearly five months after the occurrence of the heart attack. This includes (a) those men who remained unemployed throughout the year, plus (b) those who had not returned to work until 120 days or more after discharge from hospital. Considering the total population of respondents at the third stage (N=293), the following proportions of men in each occupational category were not employed at 4.7 months after the heart attack: Group 1—19 percent, Group 2—25.5 percent, Group 3—33 percent, Group 4—58 percent. This breakdown correlates with findings reported by other researchers: that cardiacs in the lower occupational stratum were unemployed for a longer period of time than were cardiacs in the upper occupational stratum (Reeder, 1956; Safilios-Rothschild, 1970; Strauss, 1966; Smith and Lilienfeld, 1971).

These figures on employment status provide some indications of the differing impact of illness on the life situations of the heart patients at one point in their posthospital experience. They are not explainable by any clear association between measures of severity of illness and occupational status. Since explanations of these data will be reviewed at a later point in the chapter, it is necessary here only to make the point of the differing positions of the patients in regard to the relative impact of illness. The fact that the proportion of semiskilled and unskilled workers still not back at work was three times larger than that for the executives and professionals implies that there are some additional aspects of life experience, problems, and opportunities which distinguished the two groupings. These will be reviewed later in the chapter and will be considered in more general terms in Chapter 10.

These data on work return can be viewed in the context of reports by other researchers on the same issues. Simple comparisons of findings from other studies cannot be made with the data in this volume, however, given the differences in characteristics of study populations, study design, and research methods. Since the men in the study population reported on here were selected in part on the basis of a "clear" health history prior to the first hospital admission, this group at the outset differs substantially from other heart patient populations whose work history has been investigated.[9] While the criteria for inclusion of patients in the study population vary among the differing investigations, it appears that there is a general finding of high proportions of men back at work one year after a first myocardial infarction. The range is generally between 70 and 95 percent, depending on the nature of the occupation, age of patient, previous condition, and other variables. In a large, relatively recent study of men with first myocardial infarction, Shapiro, et al., report that nearly 90 percent of men who left the hospital had returned to work as of 12 months after the infarction. There was some variation by age and occupational status: 93 percent of the white collar workers and 85 percent of the blue collar workers were back at work. The more favorable data on work return was reported for younger men.

Work Return and Changes in Plans

Of the men who returned to work during the year, a sizeable minority initially went back to their jobs on a full-time basis (37 percent). As Table 5 shows, however, the pattern of return varied by occupational type, and considerably higher proportions of Group 4 returned on a full-time basis than did those in other categories, particularly white collar workers. This finding may be linked to the trend reported earlier regarding date of return to work. Higher status occupational groups returned earlier and were able to ease in through initial part-time employment, while higher proportions of blue collar workers stayed out until they were able to undertake full-time work.

While they were still in their hospital beds, most patients planned on returning to the same place of work. At T_3 the cohort was examined in terms of actual patterns of initial return. Within the population as a whole, we found virtually the same proportions as anticipated at T_1. Thus, 79 percent of the patients had gone back to the same place of employment, 9 percent of the respondents had returned to a different place of employment, and the remainder were unemployed.

If we consider only those who actually returned to work, we find that as many as 90 percent of the study population at T_3 were at the same job, with no significant differences among different occupational groups. Perhaps a more important aspect of return to the former employment is the issue of change in type of work. As may be seen, 73 percent of the T_3 group reported doing the same type of work as before they became ill. These

Table 5. Work Experience During Study Year. By Percent Within Occupational Group.

	Percent of Cohort "Yes" Response	Percent Giving "Yes" Response Occupational Group			
		I	II	III	IV
Total T₃ Cohort:					
Has patient worked during previous year.	87.7 (257)(293)	98.3 (57)(58)	92.9 (91)(98)	88.9 (48)(54)	73.5 (61)(83)
Returned to same place as pre-illness.	78.5 (230)(293)	89.7 (52)(58)	86.7 (85)(98)	77.8 (42)(54)	61.4 (51)(83)
Employed During Year:					
Initially full-time upon return to work.	37.4 (96)(257)	33.3 (19)(57)	24.2 (22)(91)	41.7 (20)(48)	57.4 (35)(61)
Initial return to same place of work.	89.5 (230)(257)	91.2 (52)(57)	93.4 (85)(91)	87.5 (42)(48)	83.6 (51)(61)
In Main Employment:					
Same type of work as before illness.	73.0 (187)(256)	86.0 (49)(57)	83.3 (75)(90)	70.8 (34)(48)	47.5 (29)(61)

proportions were highest in the white collar categories. Of interest, however, is the fact that a little less than half of the semiskilled workers were doing the same work as before. Thus, while the majority of those reemployed returned to the same location and the same job, the actual work picture was appreciably different for the blue collar workers. Reeder has also reported that a larger proportion of cardiacs in manual occupations were compelled to change jobs, in comparison to those in nonmanual occupations (Reeder, 1956).

Health considerations apparently played a major role in inducing these changes. Among those employed patients who changed jobs, virtually all indicated that their new job involved either less stress and responsibility or less physical exertion. Further, approximately four-fifths of the changers also indicated that the changes had been made for health reasons, either in whole or in part.

Illness and Its Consequences at Work: A Review of Problems

PROBLEMS DURING EARLY PERIOD.   As we have seen, patients from the various occupational categories went back to work at different rates, and some returned to full-time work while others began on a part-time basis. A large minority (40 percent) reported that they had problems associated with the illness during the initial period after work return. In the reporting of problems there were no differences between patients from the different occupational groups. Nor were there differences between those who initially returned full-time or part-time. *Date* of work return was not associated either with the presence or absence of reported problems.

Among those who reported difficulties in the first period after return to work, some common problems of adjustment tended to emerge. The problems reported appear to center on concerns of competence, health symptoms, and the obstacles posed by the illness and the therapeutic regimen. The difficulties reported, in order of frequency, were: (1) occurrence of fatigue and other physical symptoms (23 percent), (2) problems in adjusting to reduced physical activity (18 percent), (3) conflicts between the demands of the job and the requirements of therapy (15 percent), (4) concern about adequacy in performance (12 percent), and (5) problems in coping with job pressures and tensions (10 percent). These items were coded on the basis of their being initial responses to an open-ended question and they indicate saliency rather than a systematic tapping of each area.

Current Problems at T_3

When asked the same type of questions regarding their *current* problems at work, the employed men reported in substantially lower proportion on difficulties associated with their heart condition. Thus 14 percent of those employed at T_3 reported difficulties at work at one year, in contrast to the 40 percent who had reported difficulties after their initial return to work. The more important finding, perhaps, is the obverse side of the percentage: namely, that at T_3 86 percent reported no work problems associated with the heart condition. This figure must be considered in terms of the fact that it refers *only* to those employed, and that a proportion of the original cohort had either never again worked or were, at T_3, unemployed mainly because of health reasons.

   Within the working group who reported problems at T_3, the order of magnitude was somewhat different from that of when they first returned to work. Thus, the highest proportion of responses at T_3 centered around adequacy of performance: they were concerned that they

were not able to carry out their work role as well as
before the illness. Next in rank was the conflict between
the requirements of the therapeutic regimen and those
of the job, particularly in regard to strenuous types of
physical activity. It is significant that the problem of
fatigue and physical symptoms, while of first rank earlier, was noted by only one employed man at T_3.

Problems at Work: Experience after Early Predictions

A relatively large proportion of men who returned to
employment reported that their illness had had an
adverse effect on their work during the course of a year.
As may be seen in Table 6, the larger proportions
appear in the blue-collar group, although nearly 40 percent of the men in white-collar categories responded in
the affirmative as well. Over one-third reported that the
illness had had a negative effect on their earnings, with
the proportions differing according to occupational level.
While 30 percent reported a belief that the illness had
affected their opportunities for advancement or promotion unfavorably, there were no significant differences by
occupational level. Finally, as the table shows, a relatively
small proportion of those reporting indicated that the
illness had led to problems in their relationships at work,
either with employers or with fellow workers (13 percent). While there are some variations in proportions
when occupational levels are compared, these are not
significant.

The data in Table 6 may be compared only in crude
fashion with those in Table 3, since the two populations
are not the same size at both points in time. Viewing the
patterning of responses from the cohort at T_3 in relation to T_2, marked similarities appear between the initial
anticipation and the later retrospective perception of
reality. Perhaps most notable, however, are the data con-

Table 6. Reported Perceptions of Effects of Heart Attack on Work During the Past Year.
By Percent Within Occupational Groups. At T_3.

	Percent of Cohort "Yes" Response	Percent Giving "Yes" Response Occupational Group			
		I	II	III	IV
Heart attack had effects on work.	44.9 (123)/(274)	37.9 (22)/(58)	38.9 (37)/(95)	44.0 (22)/(50)	59.2 (42)/(71)
Negative effects on earnings.	36.5 (99)/(271)	26.3 (15)/(57)	28.3 (26)/(92)	42.3 (22)/(52)	51.4 (36)/(70)
Negative effects on promotion or opportunity for advancement.	29.8 (71)*/(238)	29.2 (14)/(48)	28.6 (24)/(84)	25.0 (11)/(44)	35.5 (22)/(62)
Effects on relationships with employer and co-workers.	12.9 (30)*/(233)	16.0 (8)/(50)	9.5 (8)/(84)	6.5 (3)/(46)	20.8 (11)/(53)

* Percentage is based only on number of men employed during the year, with "Don't know" responses omitted. Responses of men who were either self-employed or were not employed at the time of the interview were omitted.

cerning perceptions of effects on salary or earnings. Here higher proportions of blue-collar workers at T_3 report negative effects, as compared with their expectations at T_2. It is to be emphasized here again that the semiskilled and unskilled group suffered most; in this case, they claimed the most serious losses of earnings. At the same time, nearly one-half of these workers reported no negative effects on earnings as a result of the illness. Similarly, reviewing the data in each cell of Table 6, it would appear that the majority perceived and reported no problem in the areas covered. Recognition of this pattern concerning the total population does not minimize, of course, the dimensions of problems in that portion of the cohort which did report difficulties.

Other evidence drawn from responses to direct questions serves to underline the apparent differential impact of the illness upon men from the four occupational categories. Although the economic costs and their effects will be treated in greater detail in the next chapter, some brief details can be noted here. For example, men were asked in the T_3 interview whether they had lost income from work because of illness. In response to this question, 55 percent of the men reported that they had. A statistical association between income loss and occupational category became evident, with Group 4 reporting in the highest percentages (80 percent, in contrast to 29 percent in Group 1). Further, among those reporting the highest loss ($3,000 or more during the year), the semiskilled and unskilled ranked first. Thus, 40 percent of the Group 4 men had income losses at or above the $3,000 level, while of the three other groups the proportions reporting such loss ranged from 17 to 22 percent.

In light of the higher financial impact of the disease reported by men from lower socioeconomic levels, it is perhaps not surprising that significantly higher proportions of them expressed dissatisfaction with current earnings at T_3. Patients were asked to indicate on a fixed-alternative item, how satisfied they were with the amount of money they were earning. Of the men currently employed, 30 percent indicated that they were either dissatisfied or very dissatisfied. Here again, however, there was marked variation in this response by occupational level. Differential dissatisfaction with current earnings was revealed by the following percentages of employed men: Group 1—14.5, Group 2—30, Group 3—33, Group 4—45.[10] This difference in satisfaction with earnings cannot be ascribed definitely to the effects of the heart attack, since we may be observing the continuation of a pattern existing before the illness.

To what extent were early anticipations of the negative impact of the illness upon work life fulfilled? The responses of men at the T_3 stage were consistent with their earlier responses. In Table 7 percentages are presented on two major subgroups within the study population.

The first column in the table refers to those men who foresaw problems and whose pessimistic approach was later fulfilled. The second column refers to those men who had anticipated no problem but who at T_3 reported that they had experienced difficulty. The table excludes those men who responded "don't know" at one or both stages.

As the first column in Table 7 shows, on three of the four items the pessimistic predictions were fulfilled for the majority. Only in the area of interpersonal relationships was there less difficulty than had been anticipated. The second column indicates no massive problems for the men who initially gave optimistic responses.

The data do not permit conclusions to be drawn concerning the basis for accuracy of these predictions.

Table 7. Optimism - Pessimism in Predictions and Outcome.
T_2 Prediction Compared with T_3 Report. In Percent.
Only Patients Employed at T_3 Included.

	Pessimism at T_2*, Fulfilled at T_3	Optimism at T_2** Pessimism Reported at T_3
Heart Attack: Effects on Work	68.0 (68) (100)	22.9 (30) (131)
Negative Effects on Promotion and Advancement	78.8 (26) (33)	17.3 (28) (162)
Negative Effects on Earnings	64.0 (32) (50)	24.3 (45) (185)
Negative Effects on Relations with Employer or Co-Workers	29.6 (8) (27)	9.5 (17) (179)

* The percentage consists of those patients who reported the possibility of negative effects at T_2 (denominator) and those in this group who actually reported negative effects at T_3 (numerator).

** The percentage consists of those patients who reported a prediction of no negative effects at T_2 (denominator) and those in this group who reported negative effects at T_3 (numerator).

For example, accuracy may have been based upon knowledge of the situation and prospects at work, or it may have been due, in part, to a self-fulfilling prophecy. Whatever the explanation, it is clear that those men who had anticipated difficulties did, in fact, have them.

WORK AS AN ETIOLOGICAL FACTOR:
CHANGES IN PERCEPTIONS AND ACTIVITIES

Perceptions of Work in Etiology: The Background of Planning

How do these men feel about their work as a factor in causing their heart attack? What is the context within which they made their decisions on work while still lying in their hospital beds and during their post-hospital rehabilitation?

At the time of the T_2 interview, one month after discharge from hospital, the patients were asked to rate a series of factors in terms of their importance as causes of the heart attack.[11] Among these were two dealing with differing aspects of the work dimension: physical labor and emotional tension at work. The more commonly given response was work tension, with 65 percent of the 345 patients rating this as important. In response to another question, half the patients (52 percent) indicated that working too hard physically was important as a factor in the etiology of their illness.

Examining the data on the two responses together, it appears that 80 percent reported that either one or both of these factors was important. When occupational groups were compared, it appeared that executives and professionals were more likely to cite emotional stress as important. Proportions in each occupational category indicating this factor as important were: Group 1—76 percent, Group 2—75 percent, Group 3—57 percent, Group 4—51 percent.[12]

Blue-collar workers, particularly the semiskilled, cited physical exertion at work in higher proportions than did the executives, professionals, and other white collar men. Here the proportions were as follows: Group 1—34 percent, Group 2—45 percent, Group 3—56 percent, Group 4—69 percent.[13]

Work and Etiology: Views at One Year Post-Infarct

After a year, patients had had many months to reflect upon what factors had led to the heart attack. At T_3, the conceptions reported at T_2 still remained prominent. In regard to physical overwork as an etiological factor, 52 percent of the men rated it as important. This percentage was exactly that reported by the cohort at T_2. In regard to emotional tension at work, there was an increase in the percentage of men rating it as important: 75 percent at T_3, as compared to 65 percent at T_2. The main increment appeared in the blue-collar occupational levels. Whereas they had previously given emotional tension a lower rating than had white-collar workers, at T_3 a significant number assigned it greater importance than before. At the same time, blue-collar workers continued to rate physical labor as important in causing their heart attack.

One of the more significant aspects of these ratings was that at T_3 86 percent of the cohort rated either one or both work factors as important in causing their heart attack. The fact that so many held this belief at both T_2 and T_3 bears many implications for planners of therapeutic programs, for employers, and for patients themselves, as will later be seen. Given the nature of current Workmen's Compensation laws, this view means that this study population, at least, had pinpointed areas of causation in which some might attempt to make claims for compensation for cardiac injury (Hellmuth et al., 1966).

Stress at Work: Perceptions and Change

In view of the pattern of beliefs among patients regarding the role of work in causing their heart attacks, it is also useful in this review of the natural history of the illness to examine their perceptions of stresses on the job. The data are derived from responses to a series of questions used by Scotch and Levine, and adapted from other research, such as the Midtown Manhattan Study.[14] At the T_2 stage the following questions were asked:

"Now we are interested in how you generally felt at the end of an average day in your regular line of work before you became sick.
  A. Did you often feel very pressed for time?
  B. Did you often have a feeling of dissatisfaction with your work?
  C. Did your work often upset your digestion or sleep, or upset your health in any way?
  D. Did your work often stay with you so that you were thinking about it after working hours?"

The same questions were also asked at T_3 of those patients in the cohort currently employed. Thus, it is possible to compare reported perceptions at two points in time.

In addition, two questions derived from Reeder[15] were asked. These relate to level of tension experienced and to the patient's description of his own emotional state. These questions are not directly centered on work, but they deal with dimensions relevant to understanding the stresses experienced by patients in connection with their employment. Patients were asked to indicate how well each of the following statements described them: (a) "There is a great deal of nervous strain associated with my daily activities" and (b) "In general, I am unusually tense and nervous." Patients who reported that the statements characterized them either "very well" or "fairly well" were coded as giving an affirmative response. Those who responded, "not very well" or "not at all" were coded as giving a negative answer. (Discussion of the responses to these questions appears later in another context in Chapter 8, where we consider the findings in relation to data from the Framingham Heart Study population).

Discussing first the four questions which deal directly with work, several main points can be made about the data appearing in Table 8.

As Table 8 shows, concern about work after hours ranked first in terms of proportion of affirmative responses. At the other end of the range, it may be seen that one-third of the employed respondents expressed feelings of frequent dissatisfaction with work, and about one-third believed that before their illness their work had had an adverse effect upon their health. Further, for three of the items, notable relationships between work concerns and occupational status appear in the responses describing the pre-heart attack work situation. Thus, there appears a positive relationship between occupational status and (a) the feeling of being "pressed for time," being concerned with the effect of work upon health, and (c) thinking about work after hours. Looking at percentages, one may see that the proportion of executives and professionals (Group 1) was approximately twice that for men in the unskilled blue-collar group (Group 4).

At the time of T_3 the proportions of affirmative responses to all four questions had declined, although on three of them from one-fourth to one-third of employed men gave affirmative responses. The drop in the proportion of responses indicating stress and tension associated with the job is reflected in the data when individual occupational groups are compared as well. At T_3, furthermore, the linear relationships between the stress responses and occupational groups are not as clear-cut as the data concerning the pre-heart attack period, except

Table 8. Perceptions of Work Stress at Two Stages. Previous to Myocardial Infarction as Reported at T_2. Currently as Reported at T_3 by Employed Patients. T_2 and T_3 Cohorts. "Don't know" Responses Omitted.

		Percent of Cohort "Yes" Response	Percent Giving "Yes" Response Occupational Group				"p"
			I	II	III	IV	
Think about work after hours	Pre-illness	50.3 (171)(340)	77.0 (47)(61)	50.8 (61)(120)	46.7 (28)(60)	35.4 (35)(99)	.001
	T_3	37.6 (92)(245)	63.6 (35)(55)	40.9 (36)(88)	23.9 (11)(46)	17.9 (10)(56)	.001
Pressed for time	Pre-illness	45.2 (154)(341)	59.7 (37)(62)	54.2 (65)(120)	40.0 (24)(50)	28.3 (28)(99)	.001
	T_3	27.6 (67)(243)	41.8 (23)(55)	28.7 (25)(87)	11.1 (5)(45)	25.0 (14)(56)	.01
Work affects health	Pre-illness	34.1 (115)(337)	41.0 (25)(61)	40.7 (48)(118)	33.9 (20)(59)	22.2 (22)(99)	.05
	T_3	16.4 (40)(244)	24.1 (13)(54)	20.5 (18)(88)	6.5 (3)(46)	10.7 (6)(56)	.05

		Percent of Cohort "Yes" Response	Percent Giving "Yes" Response Occupational Group				"p"
			I	II	III	IV	
Frequently dissatisfied with your work	Pre-illness	33.7 (115/341)	35.5 (22/62)	34.2 (41/120)	40.0 (24/60)	28.3 (28/99)	NS
	T₃	25.1 (61/243)	32.1 (17/53)	23.9 (21/88)	15.2 (7/46)	28.6 (16/56)	NS
Nervous strain	Pre-illness	56.3 (193/343)	71.0 (44/62)	57.5 (69/120)	47.5 (29/61)	51.0 (51/100)	.05
	T₃	41.7 (120/288)	62.1 (36/58)	41.2 (40/97)	32.1 (17/53)	33.7 (27/80)	.01
Tense, nervous	Pre-illness	48.4 (166/343)	59.7 (37/62)	42.5 (51/120)	41.0 (25/61)	53.0 (53/100)	.10
	T₃	40.6 (117/288)	50.0 (29/58)	33.0 (32/97)	43.4 (23/53)	41.2 (33/80)	.20

for one item: "thinking about work after hours." In sum, while there was a general reduction in positive responses about stress at work at T_3, in most of the occupational groups from one-fifth to two-thirds of the men continued to report stresses.

Turning to two general items describing "stressful daily activities" and "feelings of tension," it can be seen that on both items about half the patients responded in the affirmative when characterizing their pre-illness state. Although there was a reduction at one year later, two-fifths continued to answer the question in the affirmative. There are differences in percentage of "Yes" responses among occupational groups, but with one exception these are not linear. In general, it can be seen that the percentage of executives and professionals tends to be higher than that for other categories, as far as "Yes" responses are concerned. The difference between Group 1 and the other occupational categories is most marked in the report on nervous strain associated with daily activities as of the T_3 stage. Here nearly two-thirds of Group 1 reported current stressful activities, while one-third of Groups 3 and 4, the blue-collar workers, did so.

Thus, these data on the whole can be viewed in terms of two principal themes: (1) that various indicators of work-related stress and tension have been reduced over the course of the year, and (2) that for sizeable proportions of men in each of the occupational groups, the presence of reported stress continued at year's end. Further, in this series of questions, although the findings are mixed, the "executive-professional" group emerges as the one with the highest proportion of affirmative responses overall. As we have shown earlier, high proportions of the men in the study population considered that work was an important etiological factor in the development of their first heart attack. Hence, we are able, through these data on continuing work stresses, to gain some indirect insights into the life style and daily situations of many men in the study group as they go back into stressful work situations.

While the data in Table 8 present percentages for the cohorts as a whole and for specific occupational groups, they do not indicate the patterning of changes in perceived work stresses among individuals. For this purpose, the data in Table 9 may be useful. Considering only those employed men who responded at both stages, Column 1 of the table shows the percentages indicating stability in affirmative response from the T_2 to the T_3 stages. The denominator is the number saying "Yes" in regard to the pre-morbid condition, and the numerator is the number saying "Yes" at the T_3 stage. Column 2 reports on the group who changed, i.e., those who originally maintained that the item did not hold for their own work situation before illness, but who now affirmed it to be true in regard to their current employment.

As the first column in the table shows, in regard to all four questions, from approximately one-half to one-quarter of the men still reported or perceived work tension over time. However, these data also reflect a marked reduction in perception of stress, with relatively large percentages of respondents no longer perceiving job stresses. Thus, regardless of the real work situations of these men, one year after the heart attack they perceive their current jobs in a different way with most reporting less stress than before. These results may be due to differences in perception and evaluation over time. They may also be attributable to the deliberate efforts of the subjects to reduce responsibilities and tensions on the job, to work in new locations, and to adopt other means of lowering physical and emotional loads. It is also evident that a sizeable minority still felt various anxieties and dissatisfactions associated with their work.

Table 9.   Continuities and Change in Measures of Reported Stress.
Report of Pre-Illness Condition Compared with Report at T_3
for Selected Segments of Cohorts.   In Percent.

	"Yes"* T_1, T_3	"No" at T_1** "Yes" at T_3
Pressed for Time	44.7 (51) (114)	12.5 (16) (128)
Frequently Dissatisfied with Your Work	44.2 (38) (86)	14.1 (22) (156)
Work Affects You Physically	26.1 (23) (88)	10.5 (16) (153)
Think About Work After Hours	51.6 (66) (128)	20.9 (24) (115)
Nervous Strain	53.0 (88) (166)	26.4 (32) (121)
Tense, Nervous	61.5 (83) (135)	22.4 (34) (152)

* The percentage consists of those patients who reported "Yes" concerning
pre-illness condition at work (denominator) and those who reported "Yes"
concerning condition in present work (numerator).

** The percentage consists of those patients who reported "No" in regard to
pre-illness condition at work (denominator) and who reported "Yes" in
regard to current condition at work (numerator).

The table excludes those who were not employed at the time of the T_3
interview.

The questions on "nervous strain in daily activities"
and on "feeling generally unusually tense and nervous"
display a pattern similar to that of the work questions.
The responses, perhaps, are more marked. In both
cases, more than half the patients reporting stress
responses before the heart attack continued to do so at
T_3. In addition, one-fourth of those who had previously
responded in the negative with regard to the pre-heart
attack stage at T_3 reported that the statements now

described them "very well" or "fairly well."

Physical Activity at Work: Perception and Change

There were marked changes over the course of the study year in regard to reported physical activity. At the time of T_2, employed patients were asked to indicate the amount of lifting, sitting, and walking that they did at work.[16] As Table 10 shows, at least 32.5 percent responded "frequently" to a question about lifting at work.

At the time of the T_3 interview, however, the pattern reported by the cohort was distinctively different from that of the T_2 interview. Frequent lifting declined drastically, with only 8 percent of the study group reporting this activity. Further, the proportions dropped in all occupational categories. The greatest percentage difference in the two responses was with Group 4, the semiskilled and unskilled workers, where the percentages changed from 54 percent at T_2 to 16 percent at T_3. The pattern of change is reversed, however, with regard to the frequency of sitting at work. This reversal occurred in all occupational groups. With respect to walking while on the job, the proportions are essentially similar at T_2 and T_3. These data may be due to trends described earlier: deliberate efforts on the part of patients to change their activity on the job. The basis for these changes is linked in part to medical advice and in part to convictions by patients that physical stress had led to the initial heart attack. Thus, such data on amount of activity, taken as a whole, reflects effort at rational change, at least in the physical sphere, for preventive and therapeutic purposes.

Table 10. Physical Activity at Work. Cohorts at Two Points in Time. Before Illness and at T_3. In Percent. Employed Men Only.

	Percent of Cohort "Yes" Response	Percent Giving "Yes" Response Occupational Group			
		I	II	III	IV
Before Heart Attack*	N = 240	N = 43	N = 84	N = 43	N = 70
A. Lifting: Frequently	32.5	9.3	26.2	32.6	54.3
B. Sitting: 50 percent or more of time on job	37.5	7●.7	42.9	18.6	18.6
C. Walking: 50 percent or more of time on job	55.4	34.9	56.0	58.1	65.8
At T_3	N = 245	N = 55	N = 88	N = 46	N = 56
A. Lifting: Frequently	8.2	●.6	6.8	6.5	16.1
B. Sitting: 50 percent or more of time on job	54.7	7●.5	52.3	47.8	44.6
C. Walking: 50 percent or more of time on job	50.6	3●.5	55.7	52.2	57.1

* These questions were added after the interview program had already begun, and hence responses are available for 240 men, or 70 percent of the population, rather than the total cohort at the T_2 stage. The same questions were asked at T_3, the respondents including all in the study population at the time. To emphasize the fact that the cohorts differ in size, the T_2 and T_3 responses are reported separately as blocks in the table, rather than as alternate responses.

HEALTH LEVEL AND WORK PERFORMANCE

Throughout this chapter we have been reporting on various dimensions of work experience of the cohort of heart patients over the course of a year. The primary analytic classification has been the occupational group, since it enables the examination of differential experiences of men with different life styles and socioeconomic statuses. We must remember, however, that while these men entered the study on the basis of relative homogeneity in health history, this situation changed during the year. As we saw in Chapter 2, some were rehospitalized, others were not rehospitalized but had symptoms indicative of significant disease process, and still others were sufficiently well so that they could not be classified into either of the two preceding categories.

What is the relationship, therefore, between health level and illness experience and the work experience of the men in the study population? How critical is health as a determinant of performance on the job in the first year after infarction?

Many physicians have seen heart patients with severe impairment who returned to work as soon as practical and undertook their jobs at full steam. Some have also seen patients with minimal physiological damage who treated themselves as if they were severely impaired, gave up working, retired to the sidelines and became long-term invalids. Though a large body of clinical and common sense experience indicates that health level is not an overriding determinant of employment experience and performance, its apparent influence must nevertheless be examined here as a pertinent part of this exploratory effort.

Questions concerning the association of health level and work may be divided into two major subcategories. Briefly put, these are that: (1) work pattern and performance influence health level, i.e., that after discharge from the hospital following a first myocardial infarction, the subsequent health of a patient is related to type and conditions of his work, and (2) that health level determines work pattern and performance. Both of these can be examined in an exploratory fashion through review of data collected from the study population.

In regard to the first subquestion, it is useful to recapitulate here the data reported in Chapter 2. In that chapter, an extensive review was described in which efforts were made to determine variables significantly related to rehospitalization, death, and health level throughout the year. Included in that review were a number of variables related to work, including those which dealt with conditions and situations before the heart attack as well as those which existed during the study year. No association of the rehospitalization and health variables and the work variables was found.

This does not mean, of course, that work did not play a role of etiological significance. It indicates the lack of significant statistical association between the variables employed in this study in regard to these particular indices on work and etiology. Perhaps the more significant finding, as reported in the present chapter, is that many of the men *believed* that work was significant in causing the heart attack and that many acted as if it were and changed their work activities and employment in various ways.

The second subquestion, in contrast to the first, regards (a) health level as the independent variable, and (b) work pattern and performance as the dependent variable. In order to explore the question, the variables on work reviewed in this chapter were examined in relation to measures of health level.

For the purposes of this examination, a select population was drawn from the total study group. This consisted of men on whom there was information from their physicians at T_3 rating health level and reporting rehospitalization experience. This group was classified into three categories: (1) rehospitalized during the course of the study year for heart-related illness, (2) not rehospitalized but reported by the physician as having developed significant additional illness or symptoms, and (3) those reported by their physicians as having been "well" during the year. (These categories were discussed in greater detail in Chapter 2.)

As the analysis proceeded, it became apparent that on responses concerning work, the differences between categories 2 and 3 (the "symptoms" and the "well" groups) were of a minor nature. Hence, for our brief review here we combine these two groups, referring to them as the "Nonrehospitalized" (N-R). They can then be compared with the first group, the "Heart-Rehospitalized" (H-R).

In terms of work experience, those who were rehospitalized for heart-related causes during the year (H-R) differed in a number of respects from those not rehospitalized. Some of these differences might be predictable. At the time of T_3 a higher proportion of the heart-rehospitalized were currently unemployed. In fact, 44 percent of this group were not working, while only 10 percent of the nonrehospitalized were unemployed. A substantial proportion of the H-R group (33 percent) did not work at all during the year; this was true for only 8.1 percent of the N-R men.

Further, as the data on employment imply, the two groups differed in their assessment of the impact of their illness on their work experience. Among those currently employed, more of the H-R group reported experiencing difficulties or problems at work as a result of their heart condition (35 percent as compared with 12 percent for the N-R men). Of the H-R group, 60.5 percent indicated various ways in which their illness had affected the nature of the work they were performing, as compared with 41 percent of the N-R men making such indications. A somewhat higher proportion of the H-R group indicated that their heart condition had affected their chances for promotion and long-term advancement (H-R: 44 percent; N-R: 29 percent). Similarly, the rehospitalized men reported in greater proportion that their illness had had a negative effect on their salary or earnings (H-R: 59.5 percent; N-R: 38 percent). One interesting aspect of this, however, is that the employed H-R men expressed higher satisfaction with their current earnings: 88 percent indicated satisfaction, while 67 percent of the N-R group did so. This finding may be a product of the lowered expectations of the rehospitalized men. Recognizing the apparent deficits and problems imposed by their illness, they may simply have been happier to be able to have earnings at all.

Further, as might be expected, those rehospitalized more often reported actual loss of income as a result of their illness than did those in the nonrehospitalized group. Consistent with this, the H-R men reported higher dollar loss. For example, 50 percent stated that they had had a salary loss of $3,000 or more during the year, while about one-fifth of the N-R group did so.

In considering the effects of illness on subsequent work experience, it should be clear that these data are referring to matters of degree, as far as the cardiac patients are concerned. All are heart patients, and the system of classification only differentiates by level of severity of illness over the course of the year. For the total population, the effects of illness upon work were not inconsiderable. But for those who had the greater burden of illness, as measured by rehospitalization, the costs were greater in terms of opportunity, problems, money and other factors.

WORK AS A RESOURCE: SOME ASPECTS AND PATTERNS

As we noted earlier, aside from its obvious economic function in the lives of these men, work provides social, psychological and institutional supports to aid their recovery. As a group, the men comprising our population had been active members of the work force prior to their heart attack, with 96 percent employed full time. Their work had been a core life activity, providing a central focus to their lives. After their illness, return to work symbolized more than the simple resumption of earnings. It was also a return to productive occupations which reinforce and restore feelings of personal competence, and which offer the benefits of daily physical activity and social interaction with peers and other associates.

Yet, in this sense of work as a resource for rehabilitation, opportunities were differentially available to men in the study population, depending on their position in the occupational scale and social class system. On the whole, white collar workers (Occupation Groups I and II) reported optimistically that they would return to the same job and to the same type of work, and actually did so in higher proportion than blue-collar workers. They had fewer concerns than did blue-collar workers with regard to their reentry into the work force, and they subsequently reported fewer difficulties at work at the end of the study year. It was apparent from the data that the blue-collar workers were seen as more expendable by employers, and the proportion remaining unemployed during the year was higher among them.

Further, regardless of occupational status, nearly all of these men perceived that stress at work—physical or emotional—contributed to causing their heart attack. Actual stress events, such as lifting heavy weights or other severe physical or emotional exertion, could in real ways affect health and hamper the rehabilitation process during the year. These aspects, however, do not outweigh the more positive aspects of work as a resource for rehabilitation.

SUMMARY

In this chapter we have examined data relevant to a series of areas pertaining to the employment careers of the patients. These were: (1) plans to return to work and possible changes in type of work and location of employment; (2) problems associated with employment after the heart attack, including loss of earnings, lack of advancement, and interpersonal problems with employers and co-workers; (3) beliefs concerning the role of work as a factor in etiology of the illness; and (4) some characteristics of the actual work return experience. In this examination three major themes in the data emerged. These were: (1) the influence of occupational status on subsequent work experience and problems after the heart attack; (2) the negative relationship of rehospitalization to subsequent work opportunity and experience; and (3) the pervasive assumption among nearly the entire study population group that work in some way was related to the etiology of the heart attack.

At T_3, on year after admission to the hospital, 84 percent of the total patient population was currently employed. Occupational status was associated with the pattern. Nearly all of the executive and professional level patients were back at work, while fully one-third of the semiskilled and unskilled men were unemployed. Most of the latter had remained out of work over the course of the study year. In addition, at T_3, executives and professionals were more likely to be working on a full-time basis than the semiskilled or unskilled.

The pattern of differentiation by occupation type was found also in rate of return to work. Among those men who returned to work, most (84 percent) did so within four months after discharge from the hospital. There was, however, a negative association between date of return and occupational status. As many as 58 percent of the semiskilled and unskilled were still unemployed at five months after admission to the hospital, in contrast to nearly 20 percent of the executives and professionals.

The association of problems at work with occupational type was evident in loss of earnings, changes in the nature of the job, negative effects on the job, etc. Here the blue-collar men reported more difficulties.

In addition to the blue collar men, a second principal group with difficulties in the work area consisted of those rehospitalized over the course of the year. As might be expected, their apparent higher level of illness was linked to their greater income loss, problems at work and limitation on promotions, as compared with those who were not rehospitalized. There was no significant statistical association between rehospitalization and occupational status. Hence, we will not correlate the fact that blue-collar workers had more difficulties with their having been particularly subject to rehospitalization. Instead, two themes emerge from the data, pointing to two sub-populations as those with particular difficulties: the blue-collar group and the men who were rehospitalized.

On one principal point, on the whole, there was no differentiation. There was general agreement that, in one way or another, conditions at work contributed to the etiology of the heart attack, whether the reference was to physical stress or emotional tension. Although white-collar men tended to cite emotional strain and blue-collar men physical strain, the net effect was that about 85 percent blamed work in one or both of these areas.

This belief concerning work had perhaps some favorable aspects in terms of personal health planning, for considerable proportions of men apparently attempted to reduce emotional tensions associated with their work. Of those employed at T_3, a lesser proportion reported physical strain as a cause of their heart attack as compared with the employed population at T_2. Most of the semiskilled and unskilled who returned to work went back to the same job, but to a different kind of work, designed to relieve the pressures and strains. Among those men who had earlier reported either emotional stress or tension at work, there was marked decline as far as reporting it on the current job at T_3 was concerned. However, given the possibilities to be gained through making claims under Workmen's Compensation laws, through lawsuits, and other avenues, the set of beliefs about work and heart disease stands as a possible threat for employers and as a possible hindrance to workers themselves in finding new employment.

NOTES

1. For a description of the system of occupational classification utilized, see Note 4, Chapter 1. Further, for purposes of brevity, "white collar" and "blue collar" as used in this chapter are as follows: "White collar" refers to Groups 1 and 2. "Blue collar" refers to Groups 3 and 4.
2. For other information on planning while in the hospital, see Croog and Levine, 1969.
3. Of the total population, 4 men were unemployed as of T_1. They comprised 1.0 percent of the study group.
4. Results may be different in periods of economic recession.
5. Chi-square $= 24.40$, df $= 3$, $p < .001$.
6. Those patients who responded "Don't know" have been excluded from the table. Their addition to the number reporting possible problems would, of course, raise the relative proportion of patients who indicated concerns, anxieties, or uncertainties about work.
7. One important factor is the difference in physical exertion which various occupational levels demand.
8. For further discussion of the employment problems of the cardiac worker and their relationship to employer attitudes, see Reeder, 1958; Reeder, 1965; Lee et al., 1957; Olshansky et al., 1955; and Warshaw, 1966.

9. For additional information, see Pell and D'Alonzo, 1964; and Shapiro et al., 1972.
10. Chi-square = 12.04, df = 3, p < .01; gamma = 35.
11. For a complete list of items which patients at T_2 rated according to their perceived importance in the etiology of their illness, refer to Notes 4-7 in Chapter 1. Reference to these perceptions of etiology and their significance appears in other publications from this study. They include: Croog and Levine, 1972; Croog, (in press); and Croog and Richards, 1977.
12. Chi-square = 18.30, df = 3, p < .001.
13. Chi-square = 20.78, df = 3, p < .001.
14. The indices of perceived stress are drawn from the Life History Questionnaire used for a study of life stress and heart disease, Framingham Heart Study. See also the Midtown Manhattan Study reports, especially Langner and Michael, 1963, p. 313.
15. The questions were derived from Leo G. Reeder, personal communication; J.M. Chapman et al., 1966 and M. Schar et al., 1973. Though the items have been used as scales, we have chosen for clarity to report on tabulations for each, rather than total scores.
16. The questions were drawn from the H.I.P. study of heart patients, and have been described by Shapiro et al. in various reports on their work. For discussion of the questions and the rationale behind them, see E. Weinblatt et al., 1968 and C.W. Frank et al., 1963.

Chapter 4

FINANCES AND COSTS:
THE INFLUENCE OF ILLNESS

INTRODUCTION

Illness Costs and Financial Resources

One of the principal areas upon which serious illness may have major negative effects is the economic circumstances of a patient and his family.[1] A patient's favorable economic situation may serve as an important element in his "armory of resources," enabling him to deal with both the material and emotional costs. This resource has its obvious limits, however. The illness may eventually deplete it through the costs of care, loss of wages or salary, and limitations on future earning capacity. Yet the effects of the illness upon the financial situations of patients vary among the subgroups in the population, and these effects change over the course of time. In this chapter we turn to consideration of the economic aspects of the illness, including the issues of financial loss, need for changes in spending patterns, effects on the employment of wives, and sources of economic support.

FINANCIAL LOSS AND THE ILLNESS

LOSS OF INCOME FROM WORK.   One of the most immediate and dramatic effects of illness upon finances is in the loss of income from work.[2] Here the costs to an individual and to his family are more conspicuously evident than in the more subtle areas such as emotional life, psychological status, or even functional physical capacity. To determine the degree of loss, therefore, patients were asked at the T_3 interview whether they had lost income from work as a result of their illness. The proportion of positive and negative responses split almost exactly at the 50 percent point. Each of these segments deserves note, for they are more than just the reverse side of each other.

Table 1.   Reported Loss of Income from Work During Study Year. By Occupational Category.   In Percent.   (N = 268)

Occupational Category	No Income Loss	$1.00 to $999	$1,000 to $2,999	$3,000 to $5,999	$6,000 or More	N
1	76.0	3.7	1.8	11.1	7.4	(54)
2	61.0	6.4	12.0	16.3	4.3	(92)
3	32.7	9.6	34.6	15.4	7.7	(52)
4	24.3	10.0	18.6	28.6	18.5	(70)
Total Population	48.8 (131)	7.5 (20)	16.1 (43)	18.3 (49)	9.3 (25)	(268)*

* N=268, due to the elimination of 25 men whose response was uncodable because of ambiguity of response or a "Don't Know" answer.

An important aspect of the picture of loss of income from work is the relationship of this variable with indices of social status. In Table 1 percentages are given for the four categories of occupational status. As may be seen, in the top occupational group, the professionals and high executives, 76 percent report no loss from illness. The proportions decline progressively, and at the semiskilled and unskilled level only about 24 percent report no loss of income. More impressive is the percentage of high losses, particularly those of $3,000 and more. Here, adding together categories in Table 1 it may be seen that there is a distinctive range in percentages from Category 1 to Category 4. In Category 1, 18.5 percent reported loss of $3,000 or more, while 47 percent in Category 4 (the semiskilled and unskilled) reported such loss. That is, the group with the least annual income under usual conditions reported the highest actual loss. The same pattern in relation to loss of income is found in the case of the education variable. The college-level men reported least loss; those with three years of high school or less reported most.

As logic might predict, those men who were rehospitalized during the year reported a higher level of loss from illness than did those who remained out of the hospital. Points of comparison between the two groups may be observed in Table 2. Combining categories in order to examine those with losses of $3,000 or more, it may be seen that 50 percent of the rehospitalized reported this level of loss, while 23 percent of the non-rehospitalized did so. Rehospitalization could result in income loss by delaying the patient's return to work, or, if he had already resumed employment, preventing him from continuing. Findings are not explainable by any high concentration of Group 4 men in the rehospitalized category.[3]

It may be that these data on loss of income as a

Table 2.   Reported Loss of Income from Work During Study Year.
By Rehospitalization Status.   In Percent.   (N = 249)

Rehospitalization Status	No Income Loss	$1.00 to $999	$1,000 to $2,999	$3,000 to $5,999	$6,000 or More	N
Rehospitalized for Heart*	35.7 (15)	4.8 (2)	9.5 (4)	31.0 (13)	19.0 (8)	(42)
Not Rehospitalized	52.2 (108)	8.2 (17)	16.9 (35)	15.5 (32)	7.2 (15)	(207)
Total Population	(123)	(19)	(39)	(45)	(23)	(249)**

* Rehospitalization category includes patients who were rehospitalized for heart disease one or more times during study year following discharge for their initial admission.

** Reduction in numbers to 249 is due to restriction of rehospitalized group to those rehospitalized for heart. In addition, 25 men were lost due to ambiguous or other uncodable responses.

result of illness reflected mainly social class differences. Those in the white-collar and business occupations were more likely to be in situations where employers could carry them during a period of serious and extended illness or where insurance was available. Since this was the first such illness for all men in the study population, the situation was less burdensome for their employers than it would have been had the men remained out of work for extended periods and multiple times. Further, some of the men in this group were owners of businesses themselves, and a number of these were able to take time off without loss of income. The situation was different, however, for blue-collar workers, particularly the semiskilled and unskilled, for whom days away from work usually means loss of income.

CHANGES IN TOTAL EARNINGS AND FAMILY INCOME.   The preceding data pertain to estimated income loss attributed by the patients to their illness. There are, however, other, less dramatic, financial consequences. At the end of the study year, it was possible to compare reported income from wages and salary with those before the illness. The data indicate that, in accordance with expectation, those men who had been rehospitalized two or more times during the year were in a less favorable position in terms of earnings than those who experienced only the initial hospitalization.

Let us look first at the population as a whole. Table 3 shows annual salary levels by quartile reported by the rehospitalized and nonrehospitalized patient populations both before illness and at one year after. Separate distributions are presented: (a) for all men according to hospitalization status, and (b) for employed men only. These quartile figures permit comparisons between the salary level frequencies of the populations as a whole. They do not, of course, show changes for individuals in income from earnings.

As may be seen, at one year the median salary level for the group of "heart-rehospitalized" patients had declined by approximately $2,000, as compared with the pre-illness figure. For the group not rehospitalized during the study period, the median salary declined by only several hundred dollars.

Further, of the men rehospitalized, salary levels at T_3 for one quarter of the men were zero, while the salary level of the first quartile for the nonrehospitalized patient population at T_3 was $5,396. There is a difference in pattern for the two groups for the third quartile, however. For the rehospitalized men the third quartile figure was markedly less at T_3 than at the pre-illness stage, but for the nonrehospitalized men, the third quartile figure was approximately the same at T_3 as it had been at the pre-illness stage. These data must be read cautiously, but they reflect the fact that the rehos-

Table 3. Salary Levels Before the Illness and at T_3. By Quartiles.

| | Rehospitalized for Heart | | | | Not Rehospitalized | | | |
| | Pre-Illness* | | At One Year Post Admission | | Pre-Illness | | At One Year Post Admission | |
	All Men	Employed Men Only	All Men	Employed Men Only	All Men	Employed Men Only	All Men	Employed Men Only
Quartile 1	$5,881	$5,881	No Salary (Unemployed)	$5,104	$6,188	$6,251	$5,396	$5,871
Quartile 2 (median)	$7,305	$7,305	$5,312	$6,667	$7,682	$7,772	$7,377	$7,781
Quartile 3	$9,066	$9,066	$7,569	$8,472	$10,322	$10,358	$10,408	$10,897
Interquartile Range $(Q_3 - Q_1)$	$3,185	$3,185	$7,569	$3,368	$4,134	$4,107	$5,012	$5,026
N**	46	46	43	30	223	220	225	207

* It must be remembered that data were obtained in the period 1965-1967.

** Differences in the size of the N at each stage are due to uncodable responses concerning salary.

pitalized population, as a whole, underwent a substantial negative shift toward reported lower earnings during the year after illness. There was greater salary level stability, however, for those who remained out of the hospital.[4]

These data point up the pattern of change in total populations at each stage, including those men who were unemployed. Another way of examining these materials to determine the impact of illness is to look at employed men only. Among those who were able to hold jobs both before and after illness, what was the structure of their salary level distributions? As Table 3 shows, the number of employed men changes from one period to another, and we are not examining exactly the same population at each stage. Table 3 shows distributions by quartiles for all employed men at two points in time.

The same pattern is evident as when we considered the total population, i.e., the quartile figures for salary level at T_3 for the rehospitalized population were more markedly different from pre-illness levels than were the figures for the nonrehospitalized group. There is some variation in general pattern, though. For employed nonrehospitalized men in the third quartile, the salary level was greater at T_3. Twenty-five percent of this population reported that they had an annual salary level of at least $10,358 during the period preceding the heart attack; at one year post-admission, 25 percent reported that they were earning at least $10,897.

From a slightly different perspective, other data indicate that at the end of a year the proportions of low-salaried men markedly increased in both groups. Among those who were rehospitalized, 13 percent earned $100 a week or less before the illness. At T_3, however, 43 percent within this group had salary incomes at this level. This decline occurred because a high proportion of these men (13 of 21) were unemployed and thus had zero income from earnings.

Among those not rehospitalized, nine percent had earned incomes of $100 per week or less before the illness. At one year, this proportion was 20 percent. The population was thus transformed over the course of the year into one in which notable proportions had either no earnings or were at the low end of the salary scale.

While data on salary are useful in reflecting the economic status of the patient, they present only a partial picture of the year following illness and the economic condition of the family as a whole. A broader view can be obtained through consideration of total family income, including funds from all sources, since other supports may cushion or perhaps even improve the situation of patients and families. These include the earnings of a working wife, the contributions of children, and money from pension or insurance sources, from gifts, loans and investments.

In Table 4 it is possible to compare the distributions of total family income at two stages, prior to the illness and at T_3. The data show that when total family income is considered, the same basic patterns are evident as were observed in regard to the patient's salary income. For most patients there are few other financial resources to offset the decline in income from salary. In the case of the rehospitalized group, nearly one-third at T_3 reported a total income of less than $5,000, while previously about eight percent did so. Among those not rehospitalized after the first event, there was also a proportionate difference between the pre-illness and T_3 stages, with six percent and 11 percent, respectively, reporting less than $5,000 per year in total income.

At the higher income levels, however, the picture is somewhat different. Among the rehospitalized there is a drop in the percentage reporting total income of $12,500 or above from the pre-illness to the T_3 stage. For those not rehospitalized, the proportions reporting

Table 4. Total Family Income for Year Preceding Illness and End of Study Year. By Rehospitalization Status.

Not Rehospitalized

Total Family Income for Year Preceding Illness	Under $5,000	$5,000–$7,499	$7,500–$9,999	$10,000–$12,499	$12,500–$14,999	$15,000 & Over	Total	Percent
Under $5,000**	(7)	(4)	–	–	–	(2)	(13)	6.2
$ 5,000 – $ 7,499	(10)	(24)	(6)	(1)	(1)	–	(42)	20.0
$ 7,500 – $ 9,999	(5)	(18)	(28)	(15)	(2)	–	(68)	32.2
$10,000 – $12,499	(1)	(4)	(12)	(19)	(1)	(4)	(41)	19.4
$12,500 – $14,999	–	(2)	(1)	(1)	(1)	(6)	(20)	22.2
$15,000 and over	(1)	(2)	(2)	–	(10)	(22)	(27)	
N	24	54	49	36	14	34	(211)*	
Percent	11.4	25.6	23.2	17.1		22.7	100.0	

Rehospitalized for Heart

Total Family Income for Year Preceding Illness	Under $5,000	$5,000–$7,499	$7,500–$9,999	$10,000–$12,499	$12,500–$14,999	$15,000 & Over	Total	Percent
Under $5,000	(3)	–	–	–	–	–	(3)	7.5
$ 5,000 – $ 7,499	(4)	(7)	(1)	–	–	–	(12)	30.0
$ 7,500 – $ 9,999	(2)	(4)	(4)	(2)	–	–	(12)	30.0
$10,000 – $12,499	(1)	(2)	(3)	(2)	–	–	(8)	20.0
$12,500 – $14,999	(2)	–	–	–	–	–	(2)	12.5
$15,000 and over	–	–	–	(2)	–	(1)	(3)	
N	12	13	8	6	–	1	(40)*	
Percent	30.0	32.5	20.0	15.0		2.5	100.0	

* N excludes patients from whom adequate income information was not available.

** 4 men were unemployed at the time of T_1 comprising 1 percent of total. Two of these increased their income as shown, to above $15,000.

income above $12,500 remain approximately the same at each stage. These data do not indicate changes in income level in the top group; the category $15,000 and above ranges substantially upward. A man may thus have an income of $40,000 per year, drop to $20,000 and still remain in the category of "$15,000 and over." It is still of interest, nevertheless, that for this nonrehospitalized group the proportion of persons at the top income level was about the same at one year as it had been before the illness. (In this group 10 percent earned over $15,000 before the illness, while a year later 13 percent did so.)

Thus, in brief, these data for the populations as a whole show that at the end of a year the median income level of both the rehospitalized and nonrehospitalized was less than it had been before the illness, and that the change was most marked for the rehospitalized. They indicate also that a relatively high proportion of those who had been sickest, nearly one-third, reported incomes during the year of less than $5,000 from all sources.

FINANCIAL LOSS AND MULTIPLE CONTRIBUTING FACTORS. These data on the economic status of patients at the end of a year following initial illness describe patterns; they do not unravel the complex array of factors which underlie them. If changes were evident at the end of a year, this does not justify easy assumptions that illness was the chief variable. It seems clear, however, that those who were rehospitalized were more likely to experience income loss and a drop in economic resources than those who were not rehospitalized.[5] More information concerning the intervening variables should be gathered, however, before the "causal" factors can be sorted out.

In considering the economic data, a brief summary of findings from Chapter 3 may be useful here. As reported earlier, patients themselves were asked to assess the effects of their illness upon their earnings. More than half (56 percent) indicated that they perceived no effect. As many as 34 percent reported negative effects, however, and three percent reported some positive effects. (The remainder indicated "don't know" or did not respond.) Hence, among an appreciable minority of patients (one-third), negative economic effects from the illness were perceived.

During the year under study various factors were operative to affect job status and earnings. Promotions, voluntary changes of position, changes in the business climate, and fortuitous circumstances are only a few of the most obvious elements which affect income level.

Within the total population of patients reporting at T_3, 52 percent (147 of 283) were in a similar salary category at the end of a year, 18 percent (51 of 283) had moved into a higher salary category, and 29 percent (83 of 283) had moved into a lower category. These data indicate only the general changes in salary level for individuals during the year; they are based on movement from one category to another, and some variations within categories are not reflected. Nevertheless, the data reflects a general pattern: about one-fifth of the patients have increased their salary level sufficiently to be noted through this system, while about 30 percent moved downward.

It is apparent, and perhaps surprising, that for a minority of patients economic circumstances at T_3 were even better than they were before their illness. In the absence of direct evidence it would be inappropriate to ascribe upward or downward changes in salary to illness, and no such simplistic implication is intended. This is not to deny, however, that the illness was a key factor in causing economic stress and deprivation to a large segment of the patient population.

Costs of Care

Another area for inquiry was the cost of care, as these were perceived by patients at the T_3 stage. Information was developed through several questions bearing on types of costs. Since some of the men were rehospitalized after the initial episode, their financial history is beclouded by the mixture of costs from the first illness with those of subsequent illnesses.

Questions in the interviews were concerned first with the cost of the initial hospitalization: "How much of your hospital bill did you, yourself, finally have to pay? What was the amount not covered by insurance and which you had to take care of out of your own pocket?" Another question probed the costs of doctors' services in the hospital during the first hospitalization, "not counting anything which may have been paid by insurance." These questions were followed by others covering the sequellae of the illness: out-of-pocket costs of medicines and laboratory tests during the year. Finally, a question dealt with the total amounts paid by the patients during the year, subsequent to discharge from the hospital.

The distributions reported in Table 5 show the various personal costs reported by patients, excluding payments by insurance. The majority of patients paid either nothing at all or a moderate amount (less than $200) for their initial hospitalization. Half reported that they paid nothing for services by physicians while in hospital, and an additional 23 percent reported costs of less than $200. During the course of the year most patients reported paying either nothing or less than $100 total for (a) medicines and prescriptions and (b) laboratory tests and electrocardiograms. Similarly, total expenses for physician care among those reporting were on the lower end of the scale.

Table 5. Estimated Personal Costs of Initial Illness According to Reports by Patients at End of Study Year. In Percent. (N = 293)

	No Reported Costs	$1-$99	$100-$199	$200-$399	$400-$599	$600 & Over	NR***	N
				Costs During Year for Patients				
First Hospitalization	34.2	13.6	7.9	16.1	8.5	12.5	7.2	293
Physician for First Illness	49.5	11.6	11.9	11.7	2.4	1.6	11.3	293
Medicines	31.5	41.2	15.0	9.2*	–	–	3.1	293
Lab Tests	54.9	28.6	10.2	2.1**	–	–	4.2	293
Medical Bills During Past Year	34.5	31.4	10.6	5.4	1.4	.7	16.0	293

* 3.7 percent (included in the figure) indicated $600 or more.

** 1.0 percent (included in the figure) indicated $600 or more.

*** NR indicates Non-response, "Don't Know," or uncodable response.

The data on medicines, lab tests, and physician services cover the full course of the year and include the total population. When those patients who were rehospitalized are removed from the group, the pattern of distribution remains generally similar. Thus, from these data as a whole it appears that the total impact of costs on the patient group was not appreciable and that the costs of care were mainly borne by other sources.

One additional feature of these data deserves note. When the distributions are examined in relation to occupational status of patients, a positive relationship between out-of-pocket costs and occupational status appears, at least in regard to some items. (See Table 6.) Looking at those who reported paying nothing out-of-pocket, it appears that for the semiskilled and unskilled both the costs of care and medical services were minimal for the initial hospitalization. The same holds for medical bills for these groups over the course of the year.

This picture of costs can be contrasted with that reported previously concerning loss of income. Though blue-collar workers had higher income losses, greater proportions paid nothing for their actual care. Those in the higher occupational levels, while reporting minimal losses, had somewhat higher out-of-pocket costs. This pattern is consistent with expectation, given the fact that higher income persons may be charged more and may elect to have additional services and private hospital rooms.

Changing Patterns of Expenditures

Among the effects of illness are changes in patterns of expenditure. In the case of the heart patient study population, data were collected concerning ways in which various types of spending patterns were altered during

Table 6.   Costs of Care: Characteristics of Those Reporting "Nothing" or "No Costs."   In Percent.*

	Percent Reporting No Costs			
	Expenses: First Hospitalization	Expenses: Care by First Physician	Expenses: Medicine	Expenses: Physician Bills During Year
Occupational Category				
1	23.2 [13]/[56]	37.0 [20]/[54]	25.0 [14]/[56]	30.8 [16]/[52]
2	30.8 [28]/[91]	52.3 [45]/[86]	30.1 [28]/[93]	32.9 [26]/[79]
3	42.0 [21]/[50]	52.2 [24]/[46]	27.8 [15]/[54]	40.0 [18]/[45]
4	50.7 [38]/[75]	75.7 [56]/[74]	43.2 [35]/[81]	58.6 [41]/[70]
Total N	272*	260*	284*	246*
Educational Category				
1 Year College or More	23.6 [17]/[72]	41.8 [28]/[67]	27.0 [20]/[74]	37.3 [25]/[67]
4 Years High School	36.9 [31]/[84]	51.2 [42]/[82]	31.0 [27]/[87]	40.0 [28]/[70]
3 Years High School or Less	44.3 [51]/[115]	68.2 [75]/[110]	36.9 [45]/[122]	44.4 [45]/[108]
Total N	271**	259**	283**	245**

	Expenses: First Hospitalization	Expenses: Care by First Physician	Expenses: Medicine	Expenses: Physician Bills During Year
Rehospitalization Status				
Rehospitalized One Or More Times for Heart During Study Year***	36.4 [16]/[44]	62.5 [25]/[40]	25.5 [11]/[43]	40.0 [14]/[35]
Not Rehospitalized During Study Year	37.7 [80]/[212]	56.4 [115]/[204]	34.3 [78]/[224]	42.1 [82]/[195]
Total N	256	244	267	230

* Percentages are based on those in each category responding "Nothing" or "No Costs." Variation in size of the N is due to elimination of those whose responses were coded NR.

** Did not use responses coded NR. Also education information on one man was not available.

*** Since only heart rehospitalized patients are included, size of N is accordingly reduced.

the year following the initial hospitalization. In the T_3 interview these questions dealt specifically with changes brought about as a result of illness, including expenditures for food and clothing and delay in payment of bills. These questions dealt with experience during the year, without reference to the present. Hence, to aid in assessing the longer term effects, patients were also asked in the interview whether they were still spending money differently than they had before their illness.

As the first column of Table 7 shows, only about one-fourth of the patients reported making changes in expenditures for food and clothing, and about the same proportion reported postponement of payment of bills because of the illness. Further, at one year about the same proportion were still spending differently than before the illness. In general, there was a reduced pattern of spending in the group which had changed. Only a small proportion (three percent) reported increases in expenditure brought about by the illness. We can view these data now from the obverse side: for the majority of patients (75 percent), it would appear that the illness (a) led to no changes in expenditure or (b) led to changes in spending which were no longer being followed at one year.

When asked about the effects of the illness upon various expenditures for wife and children, about five percent of the married patients indicated that their wives had altered their spending patterns during the year, and about three percent noted such changes in their children. While these data are drawn from open-end questions rather than a systematic query on the specific issue, it is nonetheless apparent that few patients reported marked change in expenditure habits among other members of the household as a result of the illness. One feature of the table is the relationship between occupational status and changes of expenditures, with the

Table 7. Reported Perceptions of Changes in Plans or Spending at One Year.
By Percent Within Occupational Category and Rehospitalization Status.

	Percent of Total Who Responded "Yes"	Occupational Category (N=292)*				Rehospitalization Status	
		1 N=58	2 N=97	3 N=54	4 N=83	Not Rehospitalized N=228	Rehospitalized N=45
Changes in Food and Clothes Spending	25.6	10.3	15.5	27.8	47.0	24.6	31.1
Postpone Payment of Bills During Year	24.5	10.3	15.5	33.3	39.8	23.2	35.6
Delay Hospital Bills	13.3	6.9	9.3	20.4	18.1	11.8	24.4
Spending Differently Than Before Illness	24.2	13.8	16.3	27.8	38.6	21.0	31.6

* Percent responding "Yes" within each category:

1. As a result of your illness, did you have to make changes in any way in how you spent money for food and clothing*
2. Did you have to put off paying bills or debts as a result of your illness?
3. (If "YES") Did you have to delay paying hospital or medical bills?
4. Are you spending money differently than you did before your illness?

blue-collar workers the most markedly affected.

Although common sense might inform otherwise, there was no marked relationship between change in spending and rehospitalization during the year. Though the rehospitalized group spent differently, as revealed by the various questions, the differences in percentages between the two groups were too minor to be statistically significant. The sole exception was in the case of delay of hospital bills. Though one might assume that the burdens of additional rehospitalizations would lead to significant changes in expenditures during the year, the data in this study did not support that expectation.

FINANCIAL ASSISTANCE: CALLING UPON OUTSIDE RESOURCES

AID DURING THE STUDY YEAR.   Economic problems for some patients were alleviated to some extent through outside sources. These were primarily institutional rather than family sources. To explore the extent and type of such aid, we asked patients during the T_3 interview: "In connection with your heart condition, did you (or your wife or anyone else in the family unit) receive any *income* from any kind of insurance policy or pension that paid you money during the time you were sick?" Forty-six percent of the patients responded in the affirmative.

Further, when occupational groups were compared, there were no significant statistical differences between them in regard to the receipt of such outside funds. The patients who had been rehospitalized, however, reported a higher occurrence of receipt. Thus, 61 percent of those who had been in the hospital after their initial discharge reported income from a policy or pension, as compared with 45 percent of those who had not been rchospitalized but had received such income.

Insurance was the primary source of income from outside sources. Looking at the study population as a whole (see Table 8), it can be seen that 37.5 percent of the total study population received assistance from this source. Of those receiving any income assistance, 82 percent had aid from private insurance. Other sources of assistance were Workmen's Compensation, the Veterans Administration, or some type of government pension. Only one of 293 men in this study group received income assistance from Public Welfare.

Table 8.   Sources of Income Assistance During Study Year. Institutional and Organization Sources.*

Sources of Income	Percent
Insurance Source	37.6
Workmen's Compensation	3.7
Veterans Administration	2.4
Government Pension	1.3
Welfare	.3
Other	.7
No Income From Pension or Insurance Source	53.6
No Response	.4
Total Percent	100.0
Total N	293

* Table cites first item mentioned. Since only several men mentioned more than one source, this has minimal influence on distributions.

Compared with these institutional sources of aid, it appears that help from individuals such as family members and friends was relatively small. A study of help patterns was carried out, comparing members of the kin group, friends, and neighbors in regard to the types of assistance furnished. While these materials are reviewed in detail elsewhere (Croog et al., 1972), the contributions of financial aid can be noted briefly here. In Table 9 we report on the proportions of patients who received financial help from friends and relatives. For each category, it is important to note, only those responses are included which are derived from persons with relevant kin. Thus, in regard to reporting on parents, those whose parents were deceased are *excluded* from the table. This fact of exclusion is the main reason for differences in the number of men in each category.

Table 9.   Sources of Financial Aid During Study Year Reported
from Kin and Non-Kin Sources.   Institutions and
Organizations Excluded.

Source of Financial Aid	Percent	Number Reporting*
Parents	10.4	134
Brothers and Sisters	5.8	256
In-Laws	4.2	238
Other Relatives	1.5	198
Neighbors	.3	293
Friends	3.5	287

* As indicated in the text, only those persons with relevant
  kin or non-kin are included in table. Thus, those who have
  no siblings or those whose parents are deceased are excluded.
  The number in the N column reflects this classification.

These data present a relatively clear picture. First, it is plain that the proportions reporting receipt of financial aid during the year from each category of persons is comparatively small. The most commonly cited source of financial aid was the immediate family, including parents and siblings. In-laws and friends rank nearly as high.

These brief data do not tell about the numbers who received financial aid from more than one source, however. When multiple sources are considered, it still appears that only a relatively small percentage of the total population (less than 5 percent) received financial assistance from kin or non-kin. This proportion is well below that noted earlier of those who received income from insurance or pension plans.

These data provide some clues as to the comparative supports provided by large formal organizations, such as insurance companies and government, and those supplied by individual family members, friends and neighbors. In this first major illness the primary economic resource is the individual himself, with organizations forming a second type of protection. While the kin group and friends may offer important moral support and personal services, as we indicate elsewhere (Croog et al., 1972), their financial contribution is relatively minor. Why this is so is another issue. Since resources are available, for example, the need for assistance from kin is reduced. In a culture without such resources, it is likely that the economic support role of kin during illness would be greater.

FINANCIAL AID AT THE END OF THE STUDY YEAR.   As we have seen in our description of the work experience, at the end of the year after the first admission to hospital most of the men surviving were back at work, and most were working on a full-time basis. In line with this fact, the number of men who continued to receive financial assistance at one year was relatively small. In the T_3 interview, a question was asked to determine whether the respondent was currently receiving funds from a pension or state source. In the total study population 16 percent responded affirmatively.[6]

Further, the proportion receiving these funds was

inversely associated with occupational status. Significant differences between occupational groups were found on the Chi-square test.[7] The range was from seven percent among the Group 1 occupations to 30 percent among those in Group 4, the semiskilled and unskilled.[8] As might be anticipated, those men who had been rehospitalized were receiving pensions in higher proportions than the non-rehospitalized (41 percent versus 12 percent, respectively). Though rehospitalization is not an infallible index of level of morbidity, these data indicate that the men whose year was more difficult because of illness were more likely at the end to receive pension assistance.

What was the nature of the sources of these funds? A simple tabulation sets forth the distributions among the 46 men who were receiving pension or welfare assistance. Percentages are based on the total population at T_3. Veterans' pensions ranked as the type most frequently mentioned (eight percent, or 24 men). Next were those included in the category "government pensions," which referred to all those of a Federal nature but not designated as veterans' pensions (four percent, or 12 men). State welfare was cited by two percent, or six men; a union pension was mentioned by .3 percent, or one man. Miscellaneous sources were cited by three men, amounting to approximately one percent of the total surviving and participating cohort at T_3.

These data on pensions, taken as a whole, show that at the end of the year, with most men back at work, the use of these income sources was relatively minimal. For the major segment of the study population, at least, there are few indications of retreatism or invalidism, as reflected in low reliance on pension or welfare funds. Instead, these data imply that the major groups which did receive such funds were those with higher apparent levels of morbidity during the year or those with more acute employment problems, such as blue-collar workers whose opportunities were limited. Further, nearly all those reporting pension income cited government sources of one type or another, indicating that the government plays a major role in providing support for the disabled.

Employment of Wife during Year

In times of economic stress during periods of illness, wives who have usually stayed at home may obtain employment to supplement family income. During the course of the study year, about half the wives of married men in the surviving cohort were employed at some time (N=138).[9] However, it seems quite evident that influence of the illness on the employment of wives was not substantial. In fact, by direct report of the patients, it would appear that not many wives were influenced to go to work as a result of the illness. At T_3, only 4 percent of married men reported that their wives had been employed during the study year for reasons associated with the illness.

Though it is easy to conjecture that those women who went to work after the hospitalization were those in the lower income groups who needed additional income for support, the data do not show this. Though numbers in cells are small, there appear to be no significant differences among socioeconomic groups.

Other indications that the severity of the illness did not affect employment of the wife can be seen by considering the histories of those men who were rehospitalized. Within the rehospitalized group, 18 men reported that their wives had been employed prior to the illness. This number increased to 19 in response to the question on whether the wife had been employed during the year. Finally, at T_3 the number reporting working wives was 18. The stability of these numbers over time among the group which had the most significant illness experience lends support to the hypothesis that the rehospitalization experience itself did not exert sufficient economic pressure on the wives to seek outside employment. Instead, as we have seen, other resources were employed and problems of income were met in other ways.

Finances and the Impact of the Illness: A Review of Problems

It is recognized that illness may have consequences for patients and their families well beyond the immediate circumstances of physical and emotional impairment. To ascertain the relative importance of the illness in affecting their lives during the year, several related questions were asked. One of these was phrased: "Thinking back over the past year, what have been your biggest problems?" Among the areas which were most frequently cited were those pertaining to money and those pertaining to work. The most frequently mentioned item was financial problems (23 percent), followed by work problems (22 percent).[10]

It is obvious that the two items overlap and that they should both be regarded as economic problems. For example, concerns about unemployment and finding appropriate work may be interpreted as dealing with earning a living; they may also be interpreted in terms of other meanings of work for the individual. Regardless of the interpretation of the work material, it appears that the financial dimension was a major concern for men during the course of the year.

Looking at the financial problem item alone, it appears that there is a negative association between occupational level and the citation of financial difficul-

tics. The percentages were as follows in each occupational group: Group 1: 14; Group 2: 17.5; Group 3: 24,
Group 4: 36.[11]

This inverse association is consistent with the trend
evidenced by earlier findings concerning the financial
difficulties of blue collar groups.

There was no association, however, between the
reporting of financial difficulties during the year and the
incidence of rehospitalization. Whether the patient was
rehospitalized or not, the more important variable
appeared to be the patient's occupational level, reflecting
social status, income, and resources.

In contrast to their reports about the occurrence of
financial problems during the year, many patients, surprisingly, did not foresee economic problems in the
future. At the T_3 interview, an open-ended question was
asked: "Considering your total situation at present, what
do you see as your biggest concerns or problems for the
future?" This phrasing was designed to permit the
patients to indicate areas in which they anticipated
potential difficulties. One-third of the patients did not
indicate a perception of any future problems (28 percent
answered "none," while nearly five percent responded
"don't know").

It is not surprising that the primary concern for the
future was that of survival and maintenance of health.
This was mentioned by 28 percent of the patients.[12]
Ranking close behind was the area of work as a future
problem (23 percent). Most of these 23 percent indicated
their concern about finding appropriate work in the
future, while another group expressed concern about
their capacity to carry out future work roles and to continue to remain employed. Only 10.5 percent of the
patients indicated that financial problems were a matter
for concern in the future. The majority of patients,
it is clear, made no reference to either work or finances

as possible future problems. Indeed, a substantial percentage denied the prospect of any future problems.

These data report only on the statements in interviews made by the patients themselves; we cannot assess the presence of unexpressed anxieties or concerns. In regard to the hierarchy of *expressed* predictions about problems, however, some additional comparisons can be made. There were no statistically significant differences between patients from the various occupational groups in the pattern of response about finances as a future problem. Some variation was found, however, when predictions of the rehospitalized were compared with those of the nonrehospitalized. Some 17 percent of the rehospitalized expressed concern about future finances, as compared with 10 percent of the men who remained out of hospital during the period following first infarction. While the difference is statistically significant[13], it should be noted that the percentage difference is only about eight percent.

In sum, we have attempted in this section to report on the relative impact of the illness on the finances and economic situation of patients, integrating data drawn from several open-ended questions. Perhaps the principal conclusions here are that at the end of the year there was an inverse association between occupational status and reported financial difficulties during the year. At the end of the study year, however, only a minor proportion of patients indicated any significant changes in their financial situations as a result of the illness, and only a relatively small proportion expressed specific concern about the future financial implications of the illness. Regardless of whether we are reflecting here on optimism, or denial, or on accurate assessment, these were the perceptions as reported by patients at one point in their illness careers.

Summary

This chapter has centered on several aspects of money as a resource, specifically, on problems of costs and finances as they were faced by the heart patients during the year following their entry into the study. Three major aspects were reviewed: (1) financial loss, including that involving changes in earnings and the costs of care, (2) financial assistance received from various sources, and (3) perceptions of financial problems reported by patients.

Concerning matters of financial loss, changes downward in earnings appeared as a principal trend. The condition of being rehospitalized or not rehospitalized made an obvious difference, with the former suffering the most salary loss, as well as the sharpest decline in total family income. Out-of-pocket costs of care were seen as directly related to occupational status, with those in the higher bracket having the highest out-of-pocket expenses. The pattern was counter to that reported in Chapter 3, in which those of lower occupational status fared worse in employment experience than those of higher status. Finally, an inverse relationship was found between change in pattern of expenditures during the year and occupational status; i.e., the lower income groups initiated greater changes in their spending patterns.

Nearly half the study population received financial assistance through such resources as insurance, pensions, or other aid during the study year. Since most of the men were back at work by the end of the year, the percentage of those who still received income from insurance sources, pensions, or other institutional sources was much reduced (16 percent). Compared with the number of men who were aided by these organizations or institutions, the number who were assisted by members of the kin group and by non-kin was minimal.

The impact of the illness on the employment of wives was minimal as well. While about half the wives were employed, only a small number undertook such employment as a consequence of their husband's illness.

Among those who reported having significant problems during the study year, finances and work were the problem areas most cited. The special difficulties of men in blue-collar occupations were reflected once again, as there was an inverse relationship between mention of financial problems and occupational status. Men who were rehospitalized, however, did not differ in their reports of financial difficulties from those men who remained out of the hospital. But, looking to the future, the pattern of expressed concerns was somewhat different. Prominent as perceived problems for the future were, first, survival—staying alive—and, second, being able to work. This latter item, of course, is linked to the problem of finances itself, although only a small number mentioned money as a potential future problem.

In modern mass society it is commonly held that financial support plans and assistance encourage dependency, a retreat into invalidism wherein individuals live off pensions, public assistance, and other institutional resources. In this study group, as we have seen, such support was sought only temporarily, for the most part. Further, despite the severe financial straits of some patients, there was almost no use made of welfare or other public aid funds.

NOTES

1. For reviews of the major costs of cardiac illness in both direct and indirect terms, see, for example, H.F. Klarman, 1965; Mushkin and Collings, 1959; Rice, 1965, 1966; and Smith and Lilienfeld, 1969.
2. In this chapter as in other chapters concerning income, costs, and other financial matters, the reader should keep in mind that these data are specific to the period in which they were collected. Dollar amounts cannot be used to generalize to other periods.
3. As mentioned in Chapter 3, a negative relationship was found between income loss reported at T_3 and occupation. There was no association, however, between occupation and rehospitalization (See Chapter 2). Hence, we cannot explain the higher level of loss from illness among the rehospitalized by a high concentration of semiskilled and unskilled patients in the rehospitalized category.
4. Although data concerning salary loss are considered here in absolute terms, obviously they may also be considered in relative terms as well. For example, though the income loss for higher income men could be greater in absolute terms than for low income men, in relative terms it may actually be less. The reason here would be that the dollar loss for higher income men—even if exactly equal to that of low income men—would constitute a smaller proportion of their total salary income. In this study our

other data indicate that lower income groups suffered the most income loss in absolute terms as well as in relative terms.

5. For other data on income loss and rehospitalization, see Chapter 3.

6. This figure includes those reporting receipt of disability insurance payments.

7. Chi-square = 17.52, df = 3, p < .001; gamma = .48.

8. Among men in Occupational Category 2, 8.8 percent reported receiving funds, while 18.5 percent of those in Category 3 did so.

9. This proportion of working wives is not inconsistent with the pattern of employment of women on a national level. For example, government data indicate that in 1970 51 percent of married women had been employed at some time during the year (Booth, 1973).

10. These were responses to an open-end question, and it should be noted specifically that the percentages refer to the number of men in the total study population giving that particular answer for the item. Some men also reported having problems in other areas. Hence the total number of problems cited is not indicative of the number of individuals who made responses. Other problems cited, as coded by major category were: difficulties in personal psychological adjustment to the illness—13.3 percent: concerns about reduced capacity to perform usual roles—10.5 percent: problems relating to taking proper care of themselves, avoiding situations and risks which might lead to recurrence of the heart attack—13.0 percent: the occurrence of symptoms and setbacks in health—7.1 percent. As to the number of items mentioned, 53 percent cited one, 17 percent cited two, and 4 percent cited three. Less than 1 percent mentioned four or more. The remainder of the group cited none. As the text indicates, this was an open-end question. While the listing may reflect salience, it does not constitute a systematic sampling of problem areas.

11. Chi-square = 13.36, d.f. = 6, p < .05.

12. On the issue of future problems perceived by the patients, as the text reports, two prominent items were the areas of work and, to a lesser extent, finance. Aside from these items, however, 7 percent cited problems relating to their children, mostly centering on concerns about being able to provide for them financially in the future. The major area, however, was simply the problem of survival—maintaining health and staying alive. This was cited by 27.6 percent, and thus it ranks as the first, most salient problem for the future as indicated by these men. Five percent predicted that their own lack of acceptance of the illness, their difficulty of

adjusting personally to it would persist into the future. Other problem areas cited appeared in relatively smaller percentages. As in the case of the data referred to in Note 8, some men gave multiple responses, and the percentages are therefore not to be added together as an indicator of number of individuals with problem concerns.

13. Chi-square = 6.49, df = 2, p < .05.

Chapter 5

INSTITUTIONS AND PHYSICIANS: TWO TYPES OF RESOURCES

INTRODUCTION

In the community where the heart patients in the study population lived, there were various types of professionals, agencies, institutions, and care facilities. These formed an imposing and complex array of potential supports in the "armory of resources." In this chapter we examine some of the uses of these resources over the course of the study year. The chapter first focuses on the differential levels of use of the various potential sources. It then shifts to information on the patient and his primary resource during the first year: the physician. Here we review some patterns of communication and physician advice. In the chapter which follows we examine what patients say they do about the advice and we consider the advice patterns and the compliance orientation of the patients. In the discussion we make use once again of the classification of patients by physi-

160

cians using a variant of New York Heart Association criteria (see Chapter 2).

RESOURCES AND SUPPORTS: PROFESSIONALS, INSTITUTIONS, AGENCIES

Use of Physician Services: Pattern of Contacts and Expressed Satisfaction

Of all professional and institutional resources, physicians were the most prominently and consistently used during the study year, by both the rehospitalized and nonrehospitalized patients. After being discharged from the hospital after the first heart attack patients generally maintained consistent and continuous relationships with their physicians. In the interview at one year, patients were asked whether they had a regular doctor at that time. Ninety-six percent responded in the affirmative. For the majority (84 percent) this was the same physician who had cared for them at the time of hospitalization. Since some patients were being treated by physicians in student status (residents, fellows, interns) at that time, this continuity for the population as a whole suggests loyalty to and satisfaction with their physician. The few who changed doctors had switched to an internist or a cardiologist. Only one patient described his new doctor as a general practitioner. Moreover, patients maintained regular contacts with their physicians. In their questionnaires at T_3, physicians reported that most patients (90 percent) had kept 80 percent or more of their appointments during the year.

Frequency of use of the physician varied, of course, depending upon the clinical course of the patient over the year, as well as other factors. Most patients at the time of the interview, however, had seen their physicians relatively recently. Seventy-five percent of those with a regular physician had visited the doctor within the past three months; half had visited within the month prior to the interview, in fact. Level of satisfaction and of perception of need is indicated by the fact that 90 percent of the patients with a regular doctor at T_3 said that they planned to continue seeing the same physician for care.

Further, the patients had not seen a variety of physicians for treatment or consultation during the year, despite the fact that some of them experienced additional illness and rehospitalization. In the total population at T_3, 18 percent reported having seen more than one doctor. Most of these reported contact with only one additional, aside from their original physician. Thus, it would appear that there was little switching but rather continuing contact with and loyalty to the regular physicians.

As the data indicate, the heart patients in the study had favorable impressions of the care they had received from their physicians. In the T_3 interview patients were asked, "Do you feel there are things your regular doctor might have done to help you in your recovery which he did not do?" Ninety percent of the patients had no negative comments to make on the performance of their physicians. Since the question came at the end of a year, it provides a type of perspective different from the initial euphoria which patients sometimes have concerning their physicians after they perceive themselves as having been saved from death.

Some Traits of the Physicians

Who were these physicians with whom the patients had regular contact? Some brief data on demographic characteristics and training can help to characterize them. For our purposes here, we report on the physi-

cians as seen from the perspective of the patient population, rather than as a separate group to be tabulated.

First, 52 percent of patients had doctors who were
not treating any other patients in the study group. Con-
versely, it should also be noted that nearly half the
patients in the study population had in common the fact
that they shared physicians. Whereas most of these doctors were seeing two or three patients in the study, no
group of physicians was treating large clusters of patients
in the study. Hence, findings we will present on patterns
of physician advice and doctor-patient communication
cannot be ascribed to the inordinate influence of a few
physicians on a large segment of the study group.
Approximately half the patients had doctors who had
received their medical school training in the Greater
Boston area.[1]

In general, the patients were seeing physicians who
had considerable medical experience. Half the patients
had doctors who had been out of medical school for 20
years or more. About half the patients had physicians
who were 45 years old or younger. Only five percent of
the patients had doctors who were more than 65 years of
age.

The majority of physicians classified themselves as
specialists. Thus, 62 percent of the patients had doctors
who were practicing internal medicine, while an additional nine percent had doctors classified as specialists in
cardiovascular disease. The proportion of board certified specialists is somewhat less. Doctors for 46 percent
of patients were board certified in internal medicine.
However, 54 percent of patients had doctors with no
board membership. Only about one quarter of the physicians were in general practice.

The majority of patients (82 percent) had physicians
who were engaged in full-time private practice. About 10
percent were interns, residents or fellows and about six

percent were full-time members of hospital staffs. Most patients (91 percent) were served by practitioners who were not listed as having faculty appointments at any of the local medical schools in the Greater Boston area. The remainder had appointments at Harvard, Tufts or Boston University.

Service Usage: The Clinic, the Hospital and the Physician

Aside from the physician, the hospital clinic and the hospital itself were the chief agencies for care and support during the study year. It appears that after T_2 only a minority of persons (18 percent) made use of hospital clinic facilities. The use of such facilities, as in the case of physician contacts, is characterized by high stability. With only one exception, patients going to a clinic for services indicated they had used only one clinic. The patient who was the exception reported he had visited two clinics.

The proportion making use of hospital services was slightly higher. As we reported in Chapter 2, about 25 percent of the patients were rehospitalized during the course of the study year for various causes. Aside from the physician, clinic, and hospital, however, other resources were minimally used.

Other Institutions, Agencies and Professionals

In the third interview patients were presented with a list of institutions, agencies, and categories of professionals available in the community. They were asked whether they had been in contact with any of these in order to obtain assistance. In addition, they were asked whether they had been in contact with others not listed. Within the total study group, 72 percent reported no contact and 15 percent reported contacting one. Of the remainder, seven percent reported two, four percent reported three, and two percent had contacted four or more institutional resources or professional categories of personnel.

Table 1. Distribution of Institutional and Professional
Contacts Most Frequently Mentioned.
N = 293

	Percent of Total Study Group	*N*
1 Unemployment service	11.3	33
2. Welfare department	6.6	19
3. Clergymen	5.5	16
4. Veterans' services	4.4	13
5A. American Heart Association	4.1	12
5B. Social worker	4.1	12
6. Cardiac rehabilitation clinic	2.7	8
7. Social service agency	1.7	5
8. Psychiatrist	.6	2
9. Visiting Nurse Association	.3	1

As Table 1 shows, the unemployment service and the welfare department ranked highest on the list. Clergymen ranked third, a point on which we will later comment. At the bottom of the list, eight men mentioned a cardiac rehabilitation clinic, and somewhat fewer noted contact with social service personnel. One man indicated he had been in touch with a Visiting Nurses Association.

In view of the small numbers of men who were in contact with agencies, it is difficult to make meaningful interpretations concerning variables associated with usage. For most of the categories the numbers are too small to apply statistical tests, and the percentages are based on numbers too small for extended comparison.

Some relationships appear, however, which deserve note. For example, the services of an "employment service" were most used by patients with limited recovery, i.e., those graded Class III by their doctors.[2] Those who did not have health insurance were more likely to make use of the Veterans Administration.

Use of services of one or more agencies was negatively associated with educational level, i.e., those having the least education used a greater number of services.[3] Further, those who had been rehospitalized, who lacked insurance, and who described their progress during the year as "worse than expected" were the highest users of one or more agencies. Overall, however, the total use of services was relatively small.

In sum, although the occurrence of a heart attack and the incidence of further rehospitalization and of significant symptoms made this period one of marked stress, it appears that the majority of patients dealt with their problems in other ways than through institutional resources. Among those men who were rehospitalized a second and third time, for example, it would appear that there might have been more need for services than the actual usage would indicate. Since Boston is a metropolis with the multiple resources typical of industrialized, urban areas, the low use of services deserves special note.[4]

Clergy and the Religious Institution

One resource which has rarely been examined in rehabilitation studies is the role of the religious institution and the clergy. The role of the religious institution as a source of solace and support for the patients in this study population, while difficult to measure, was probably not inconsiderable. Many of the men, for example, stated that they regarded religion as important to them in varying degrees (Croog and Levine, 1972). In the total population identified as Catholic, Protestant, or Jewish, 85 percent reported that prior to the illness they considered their religion as very important, important, or fairly important to them. Their ratings remained relatively stable over the course of the year, as did their reports on frequency of attendance at religious services.

One specific type of resource provided by the religious institution is seen in the person of the clergy. As is well known, one of the key roles of the clergy lies in linking the parishioner with the religious institution and in providing guidance and support. Yet, in the case of the heart study population, the patients were rarely in contact with clergy in regard to problems related to the illness. In fact, 94 percent reported no contact during the course of the year for purposes of help or advice.

Even given some possible error in reporting, the low incidence of contact with clergy obviously cannot lead us to assume that there were many instances of counseling and guidance. The lack of perception of the clergy as a resource in the illness (regardless of whether visits actually took place) is conspicuous. Nevertheless, though minimal contact with clergy was reported specifically in regard to the illness, the role of the religious institution itself as a resource should not be underestimated for this study population.

THE PHYSICIAN AS RESOURCE: COMMUNICATION, ADVICE, AND PATIENT COMPLIANCE

We turn now to consideration of the heart patients in relation to the key figure in their resource armory: the physician. In this section we are concerned with three principal aspects of the doctor-patient experience:

communication, pattern of advice and patient compliance with the medical regimen (Becker and Maiman, 1975; Bloom and Wilson, 1972; Davis, 1968; Francis et al., 1969; Holder, 1972; Korsch, et al., 1968; Linehan, 1966; Lorber, 1975; Reader, 1974; Rosenberg, 1971).

Effective communication between doctor and patient is vital in health care. The doctor may give clear advice, instructions or information, but often he is not heard or is not understood, or his message is retranslated by the patient. Patients, after all, can only comply with advice they have understood and accepted. Physicians often complain that some patients don't listen, or, while they may nod their heads in agreement, they either do not understand the message or have no intention of complying with it. Patients, for their part, usually have heightened concerns and anxieties, and they may fantasize that the doctor is withholding the truth from them (Waitzkin and Stoeckle, 1972). In the following discussion we will focus upon the nature of doctor-patient communication in several contexts over a span of time.

Initial Communication: Doctor and Patient at T_1 and T_2

In the interview at T_1, shortly before discharge from hospital, patients were asked, "Has your doctor discussed your case with you?"[5] Seventy-one percent stated that he had. An important feature, however, is the obverse side: nearly one-third of the patients maintained that their physician had not discussed their illness with them. The patterning in perception of communication with the physician varied by social status level. As Table 2 indicates, the lower the status of the patient, as measured by educational category, in general the less likely was he to report that the physician had discussed his case with him. In considering these findings, it is important to note that at the time of the interview virtually all the patients had been in treatment for at least two and a half weeks. Hence, in almost all cases ample time had elapsed for discussion of the case between physician and patient.

Table 2. Percentage of Men with Myocardial Infarction, at Each Educational Level, Reporting No Discussion of Illness with Their Physician in Hospital at Time of T_1 Interview.*

Educational Level	Percent Reporting No Discussion	Total Number
Total	32.0	345
Post-college: 1 or more years	8.3	24
College: 4 years	12.5	24
College: 1-3 years	25.7	35
4 years of high school	25.5	111
10-11 years of school	38.8	67
Grades 7-9	52.1	71
6 grades or less	38.4	13

Chi-square = 28.26, degrees of freedom = 6, p<.001

* As the text explains, this interview occurred shortly before discharge; on the average it was 2.5 weeks after admission to the hospital.

These findings do not simply reflect the differences between service or ward patients and private patients. While it is true that as many as 43 percent of the service patients reported that they had had no discussion of their illness with the physician, as many as 27 percent of the private patients also responded in the same way.

Controlling for educational level within the service and private groups separately resulted in the same pattern of association between education and communication at T_1. In other words, among both service and private patients, the less educated were more likely than the higher educated to report that their physicians had not discussed the illness with them.[6]

The reported lack of discussion between patient and doctor at T_1 may have been due to lack of initiative by the patient in pressing the physician for information. Of the 110 patients who reported no discussion, 68 percent stated that they would have liked to ask the physician about such matters as prognosis, future work plans, physical activities and diet. This was in response to the question at T_1, "Is there anything on your mind which you would like to ask your doctor?"

It was not feasible in this study to monitor communications between physicians and patients. Possibly all the physicians communicated fully with their patients before the first interview, and the patients' impressions were inaccurate. However, evidence from other data suggests that accounts by the patient of physician noncommunication at T_1 might not have stemmed simply from biased reporting or inaccurate impressions. For example, patients were interviewed again approximately one month after discharge from the hospital (T_2). At that time, 99 percent reported that they *had* discussed aspects of the illness with their physician. No differential perception by social status existed then in regard to whether communications had taken place.

Since all patients were able to perceive communication by the time of the second interview, it seems unlikely that some element associated with social status prevented them from perceiving it accurately one month earlier. In the absence of direct monitoring, however, we must concede the possibility that all doctors did talk to all their patients earlier, and that the relatively high percentage of reported noncommunication was the result of either inaccurate perception or unconscious denial.

Physician-Patient Communication and Occupational Plans

Among the most critical concerns of male heart patients
are the implications of their illness for employment. The
social and emotional importance of employment for men
has often been reviewed, and there is little need to
emphasize its profound meaning for masculine self-
image, family roles and patterns of social participation
(Croog et al., 1968; Friedman and Havighurst, 1954;
Morse and Weiss, 1962; Simmons, 1965). Concerns
about future work potential are important ones even
though they may not be consciously recognized or
expressed by the patient.

In the hospital interview held shortly before their
discharge, 60 percent of the patients reported that the
physicians had discussed the question of returning to
work. Perhaps equally important is the fact that at the
time of the T_1 interview 40 percent apparently did not
perceive that such communication had taken place. Possibly the physicians gave advice about returning to work,
but the patients did not perceive it as having been given.
Perhaps the physicians preferred to discuss work issues
closer to the time of discharge from the hospital. The
finding is meaningful, however, insofar as it indicates the
degree to which possible anxieties and concerns of
patients about aspects of their future employment had
been dealt with by the time of the hospital interview.

Whether they will be able to fulfill the usual
requirements of their job is a practical question of central importance to male patients, particularly those
engaged in blue-collar occupations which require physical exertion. For obvious reasons, physicians are more
likely to advise restrictions for patients doing heavy labor
than they are for patients in sedentary occupations.
When asked about the matter in the hospital interview at
T_1, patients with blue-collar occupations, as expected,

responded more frequently than white-collar workers that their physicians had indeed advised them to reduce physical exertion on the job. However, only 15 percent of all patients in blue-collar occupations reported receiving such advice by the time of the first interview.

Approximately six percent of the total group of heart patients reported that their physicians had advised them of the desirability to change jobs. All of these patients were in the blue-collar category. Within each blue-collar classification, the proportions advised to change jobs were as follows: skilled workers, 11 percent; semiskilled workers, 10 percent; and unskilled workers, 17 percent.

Perhaps one basis for suggesting job changes was the physicians' concern that patients should avoid the physical exertion of blue-collar employment.

Although many high-status patients reported that a great deal of emotional stress existed in their work and that they considered stress to be a cause of their heart attack, physicians possibly took physical rather than emotional stress more seriously as a basis for recommending a job change.

Regardless of whether the physician had given advice on a job change, at the time of the first interview a substantial proportion of patients in blue-collar occupations had either decided not to return to their former jobs or were in the process of deciding. It is important to note that not a single patient reported his intention to retire. Among 73 semiskilled and unskilled laborers, 18 percent said that they did not plan to return to the same job and 21 percent stated that they did not know if they would return. Among 46 skilled workers, nine percent stated that they would not return and 13 percent expressed uncertainty. The proportions of potential job changers were substantially lower among 128 white collar workers. Only two percent reported that they would not go back to the jobs they held before the illness and 1 percent expressed uncertainty.

It is apparent that at the time of hospital discharge many blue-collar workers had been coping with decisions concerning their employment. Some of them were clearly helped by discussions with their doctors. But it was primarily the semiskilled and unskilled (those for whom job concerns were perhaps most pressing), who reported that they had not had the benefit of physician advice and discussion up to the time of the T_1 interview.

COMMUNICATION: CONTENT AND THE NEEDS OF THE PATIENT FOR INFORMATION

These data concerning communication between patient and doctor during the period before discharge raise additional questions about patient anxieties and concerns. During the early phases of the illness and post-hospital recovery doctors communicate in many ways with their patients about the nature of the illness, advising on numerous issues pertaining to health maintenance, rehabilitation, and changes in life style. In the course of this information transmission a number of processes are going on at many levels.

The kinds of information given, the information which is not given, the way it is imparted, the time in the illness process—these are only some of the elements which affect patient response to the doctor, and, in turn, affect ways in which patients deal with their illness. For the patient, particularly vulnerable at this point, the fact of feeling uninformed or that he is regarded as some-how unworthy of the attention of his doctor, may have some negative consequences, raising his level of anxiety and stress. The feeling that the doctor is holding something back may lead to fantasies that the situation is grim, the prognosis unfavorable, and that death may come at any time. Hence, his perception of the information given links to more than the passage of information. It relates also to the quality of the doctor-patient relationship and the patient's assessment of his total situation and prospects.

Complicating the problem of understanding the patient's anxieties and concerns are various defense mechanisms, which may operate to obscure the expression of these anxieties. For example, some areas may be so sensitive or so painful to contemplate that, through the processes of repression, the patient may even be unaware that these are matters of concern. During a pre-test of the interview schedule for this study, we held interviews with a series of heart patients while they were still in the hospital under medical treatment for their illness (Croog and Levine, 1969). They were asked a series of questions designed to elicit a rating of their major sources of worry and concern. An item concerning "worry about death" was included, but surprisingly, not a single patient in the early series indicated that he was concerned about death!

These were men, it should be emphasized, who had been informed that they had had a heart attack, and were at the time in the hospital. Yet death did not concern them, or so the negative response would have us believe. Was this a valid report? Or was the process of denial at work, sweeping from awareness the awful prospect that they had literally been a heartbeat away from dying?

In this report we shall not deal with the unexpressed concerns because of simple lack of information. But this does not mean that such areas lack importance or relevance. In dealing with the *expressed* concerns, however, we are focusing on a series of dimensions which are also pertinent to recovery. They are dimensions of which the

patient is aware and that trouble him sufficiently to
mention. They also are pertinent matters for consideration in planning therapeutic programs.

*After Doctor-Patient Communication: What Does the
Patient Want to Know?*

In the treatment of cardiac illness, as in other cases of
serious disease, the advice and instructions which physicians give patients is a critical component. However, one
of the continuing problems in clinical practice is that the
pattern of communication between doctor and patient is
sometimes an imperfect one.

In the next pages we present data on the expressed
concerns of heart patients, examining their responses at
T_1 and T_2. We thus concentrate on patients in their
first encounter with illness and after they have been
under medical care for two months. We therefore take a
period during which there was ample opportunity for
perception of problems to emerge as well as sufficient
time and contacts with physicians to permit communication. As of T_1 and T_2, data are presented on the following:

1. Areas on which patients wish further advice from
   physicians;[7]
2. Social and personality variables associated with
   wanting further information from physicians;
3. Continuities between two time periods in regard
   to (a) level of medical advice wanted, and (b)
   areas of persisting concern;
4. Patterns of association of areas on which advice
   or information was wanted at two specific points
   in time.

In order to explore the possible relationships between social and psychological factors and the patient's interest in further advice and information, a series of variables were employed in cross-tabulations:[8] (a) Educational level was examined as one index of social status, (b) the Hollingshead Index of Social Position was employed (Hollingshead, 1957). (This measure is based on ratings of highest year of education and occupational level.), (c) To determine possible association of advice wanted with type of relationship to doctors in hospital, patients with private physicians were compared with those who were "service" or "ward" patients, (d) Comparisons were made between patients by age levels 30 through 39 years, 40 through 49, and 50 through 60, and (e) Ratings of traits of emotional responsiveness and control, introversion, and sociability were examined. (These were derived from a series of self-rating items developed by Burgess and Wallin which have been given wide usage.)[9] Further, we added five items regarding ambition, time-urgency and being hard-driving. These additional items have frequently been cited in the literature on coronary personality as being hypothetically related to the etiology of the illness.[10] Patients were classified in three categories in regard to each personality item, according to whether they characterized themselves as having the trait "very much" or "considerably," "somewhat" or "a little," or "not at all."

Number of Areas of Advice Wanted

An additional issue is the degree to which patients at differing stages in the early recovery process wished to have further information from their doctors, and how this might relate to social and psychological characteristics. Tabulations are reported in Table 3.

As can be seen through the percentages in Table 3, somewhat more than half the patients at T_1 and slightly

Table 3.   Number of Areas on which Patients Indicated Desire
for Further Advice or Information.   By Stage: T_1, T_2.
Percent of Total Population.

Number of Areas of Advice Wanted	Percent of Total Population T_1	Percent of Total Population T_2
0	43.8	52.1
1	24.1	23.2
2	17.1	15.4
3	9.6	6.7
4 or more	5.4	2.6
Total Percent	100.0	100.0
Total N	345*	345

* Although the original population numbered 348, three men
died before completing T_2 interviews.

under half at T_2 indicated one or more areas on which
they wanted further advice or discussion with their
physicians. At each stage most of the patients who
wanted advice specified either one or two areas of concern. Further, the table also shows that substantial proportions of patients at both interviews reported that they
had no matters on which they wanted further information from their physicians. A notable feature is the relative stability of patterns of the two time stages. Although
the problems of the hospitalization period are distinct
from those of the post-hospital rehabilitation phase, the
two stages show high similarity in numbers of areas of
concern on which patients felt sufficient curiosity or anxiety to want medical advice.

In order to determine whether desire for advice was
related to particular patient characteristics, a series of
cross-tabulations and tests of association were made.
Number of areas of advice wanted was compared with
various characteristics of the patients, including social

status, educational level, ratings on personality items, and type of status in hospital (i.e., private vs. "service" or "ward" patients). We found no statistically significant relationships.

Frequency of Citation of Items of Advice and Information Desired

Some items persisted as areas of concern from T_1 to T_2. These are recorded in Table 4 in terms of the proportions of patients who wanted information in each area.

Table 4.   Areas on which Patients at T_1 and T_2 Wanted Additional Advice or Information from their Doctors.   Rank as of T_1 Stage. Percentage Based on Total Population (345).*

Areas of Advice Wanted	T_1 Percent of Total Population	T_2 Percent of Total Population
Physical Activity	20.6 (71)	18.3 (63)
Prognosis	19.1 (66)	11.9 (41)
Work	16.2 (56)	14.2 (49)
Diagnosis	13.3 (46)	10.7 (37)
Etiology/Physiology	12.8 (44)	8.1 (28)
Diet	11.0 (38)	4.9 (17)
Therapy	5.5 (19)	1.2 (4)
Medications	3.5 (12)	3.2 (11)
Smoking	2.0 (7)	1.2 (4)
Alcohol Usage	0.6 (2)	1.7 (6)
Weight Control	--	1.2 (4)
Sexual Activity	0.3 (1)	0.9 (3)
Medical Bills	0.3 (1)	0.3 (1)

* The Table reports on the number of patients wanting advice in each area.   The tabulations reflect the fact that some patients expressed interest in advice concerning multiple areas.   The percentages, therefore, are not cumulative.

Approximately one-fifth of the patients at each stage wanted information concerning the type and degree of activities which they might perform. Further, at T_1 the highest proportions of patients wanted advice on diagnosis, prognosis and work. Specific areas which were of lesser concern were use of alcohol, weight control and smoking.

As might be expected, some variation is evident between the T_1 and T_2 periods in proportions of men wanting advice on specific issues. While general decline in percentages between the two periods appears (perhaps reflecting the fact that by one month post-hospitalization some of the men who were uninformed at T_1 had subsequently received the desired information or no longer perceived a matter as particularly salient), on virtually all items the decline in percentages is relatively small. This would indicate that some concerns were persistent. Further, such factors as educational level, age, social class, and particular personality traits did not appear to be related to a patient's interest in obtaining further information from the physician at either T_1 or T_2.

Physician Advice as Perceived by Patients

The desire for further advice from physicians is mediated by many factors, and it would be naive to assume that those patients who wanted further information were exclusively those who had not received any. For example, for various reasons patients who *have* discussed particular matters with their physicians may still want further information. Or, those who *have not* received information on particular issues may not have wanted it. The reasons for such lack of specific motivation may include the availability of such information from other professional sources or public information media, the patient's previous knowledge, his not recognizing the relevance of an area, his expectations of future communication, and perhaps, his own operating mechanisms of denial and repression.

Some perspective in regard to reported desire for additional advice can be gained by a review of content areas on which patients reported having received information from their physicians at T_2. Tabulations on percentages of patients who report receiving advice on specific topics appear in Table 5.[11]

The data in the table are comprised of those items which were reported by patients, and they can be interpreted only as indicators of patient perception and recall, not as measures of the degree to which doctors actually discussed those topics. The data, therefore, do not reflect actual need for particular types of advice, nor can they be used to indicate how well the physician appraised such need in the patient.

At the time of T_2 the items most frequently reported as having been covered by physicians concern matters of medications, diet, physical activity, smoking, and the date when the patient might return to work. Relatively few patients reported receiving advice on sexual activity, referral to agencies, or alterations in life style and living arrangements.

Review of the tabulations in Table 4 in comparison with those of Table 5 reveals some notable features. As compared with the percentages at T_2 who reported receiving advice, those wishing additional information are relatively small. The highest ranked items in Table 4 are those involving work, level of permissible physical activity, and specific aspects of the disease. Few patients wanted additional information about medications, smoking, weight control or use of alcoholic beverages. On all of these issues, 50 percent or more reported some discussion with their physicians.

Despite the reported decline in their interest in

Table 5.   Areas of Advice Discussed by Physicians as Reported by
Patients at T_2, One Month after Discharge from Hospital.
By Percent of Total.   (N=345)

Area of Advice Reported	Percent of Total Population	N Reporting Advice
Medications	89.0	(307)
Diet	89.0	(276)
Walking	79.4	(274)
Climbing stairs	77.1	(266)
Smoking	73.0	(252)
Time of work return	71.3	(246)
Weight control	65.5	(226)
Lifting things	59.7	(205)
Rest	54.2	(187)
Working part-time	51.0	(176)
Use of alcoholic beverages	50.4	(174)
Avoiding quarrels	42.9	(148)
Exercise	39.1	(135)
Nitroglycerine	31.8	(110)
Recreation	17.4	(60)
Different job: same place	14.8	(51)
Different job: new place	7.2	(25)
Living arrangements	7.5	(26)
Vacations	6.1	(21)
Sexual activity*	3.2	(11)
Future plans	2.9	(10)
Agencies - financial help	2.3	(8)
Agencies - medical care	1.4	(5)
Agencies - rehabilitation	1.7	(4)

* Cited in open-end item. Not part of initial listing at T_2.

receiving information from physicians, a large segment of the study population continued to seek information one month after hospitalization (T_2). This group included 120 men. They constitute 62 percent of those who had questions at T_1, and they are a sizeable minority within the study population as a whole (35 percent). They deserve attention as a special group insofar as they are the ones who persisted, for whatever reason, in their concerns and anxieties over the course of the recovery period.

A primary issue is why this group of patients *continued* to want information. One obvious possibility was that there were particular areas which concerned them at T_1 and which remained unresolved at the later stage.

Figure 1 reports on those patients who continued to want information on the same items at T_1 and T_2. The proportions of patients who continued to have questions on the same issues at both T_1 and T_2 ranged up to 31 percent. At T_2 the majority of the 120 patients wanted information dealing with areas other than those cited at T_1. It should be noted, however, that the numbers of patients involved are only a small percentage of the total population of patients in this study.

Figure 1

Problem Area	N at T_1	Percent of Patients Wanting Advice at T_2 on Same Area as at T_1
Activity	71	31.0 (22)
Etiology, Physiology of Heart Attack	44	27.3 (12)
Work	56	23.2 (13)
Prognosis	66	22.7 (15)
Diagnosis	46	21.7 (10)
Diet	38	15.8 (6)

Cross-tabulations were carried out in order to learn if this group of 120 patients with a continuing desire for further information differed in social and psychological characteristics from the remainder of the study population. No statistically meaningful associations were found that differentiated this group from other patients on the variables examined.

As in the case of data presented earlier, the items most frequently mentioned by the "continuing questioner" group are distinct in their relative ambiguity. They involve individual decisions by patients in such many-faceted areas as "activity" or "work," or they are concerned with the uncertainties of the disease process and the future welfare and life of the individual.

Some Features of Advice Given

In Table 5 we listed the various areas on which patients reported that they had been given advice at T_2[12]. Areas were ranked according to the percent of the total population which reported that this topic had been discussed by their physician. The percentages ranged from 90 percent downward. The most frequently noted items were those of medications, diet, and matters pertaining to exercise. Least often reported were items pertaining to use of health and social service organizations (medical care, rehabilitation, finances), the framing of future plans, and changes in living arrangements at home. A few patients noted that they had been given advice pertaining to sex activity.

No implications can be drawn from the listing that these items are equally relevant for all patients. Obviously, it is highly unlikely that a non-smoker would be given advice about smoking, or that a patient with ample economic resources would be referred to agencies for financial aid. As we have noted, the advice items were perceived by patients at a particular point in time. As such, they also reflect the physician's conception of appropriate scheduling of advice, consistent with the interests of the patient. For example, though patients may have anxiety about returning to work or concern about the financial implications, there is no general "scientific" rule that this advice should have been given earlier or later than indicated by these patients. Thus, while we are reporting on patient perceptions only, the ordering of the items by frequency may indicate more than patient needs. It may also be indicative of the physician's value systems, his beliefs about the illness and its phases, and his conceptions of the appropriate time to offer advice.

The patterning of major types of advice given, as reported by patients, derives from current conceptions of risk factors for recurrence of heart disease. For example, at one month discharge from the hospital, high percentages reported advice on matters pertaining to diet, exercise, smoking, physical exertion, and weight control. Aside from advice dealing with such specific matters, more general advice about avoiding quarrels and upsetting emotional experiences was reported by 43 percent of the respondents.

Some changes in advice reported from T_1 to T_2 should be noted. In the hospital interview (T_1), about 40 percent indicated that their doctor had not yet discussed their return to work with them. At one month after discharge (T_2), the percentage had dropped slightly: somewhat over 70 percent reported that advice on the matter had been given. Another pattern, however, remained stable: there was a relationship between advice on physical strain and occupational group at both interviews, with the blue collar workers reporting in higher proportions that they had been advised about appropriate care in lifting heavy weights.

One item at the bottom of the listing, advice on sex activity, may deserve some special note in view of its rank and its possible significance of an area of concern. As the Table 5 footnote shows, the original item was not part of the list presented to patients at T_2. Since we were interviewing husbands and wives concerning items on which there might be unpredictable and upsetting response, we took a conservative course and did not deliberately probe into their sex lives. One rationale was that negative response on the part of either husband or wife might endanger the interview and future cooperation. When they were asked if there were anything else on which they had been given advice, however, 11 patients—three percent of the total—responded that they had received advice on sexual relations.

The matter of sex activity for heart patients is one of the more difficult issues on which a physician is called upon to give advice (Green, 1975; Hellerstein and Friedman, 1970; Pinderhughes et al., 1972). A patient's seeming lack of concern is no less significant than his expression of concern. Men may be so sensitive about the issue that they may wish to avoid confronting it, and this may emerge as a conviction that this is not a problem area. The interaction of beliefs concerning the heart, male sex performance and masculine image are well known. The prospect of reduction of sex activity and the possibility of death as a result of coitus are issues on which men—and their wives as well—may have much confusion and doubt.

Was the low proportion of men who mentioned advice in this area a reflection of reality? Was this merely an artifact of the interview schedule? Was it a matter of the timing of the interview, considering that at one month post-hospital physicians might not yet have decided to advise on the topic?

Some evidence on the matter is offered by patients

in the third interview, that occurring at one year after hospital admission, as well as from the questionnaires completed at T_3 by physicians. In line with a series of questions concerning advice, the 293 patients in the third stage were asked *specifically* whether their physician had advised them on marital or sexual relations. Twenty percent answered in the affirmative.

On the other hand, a somewhat higher proportion of physicians at T_3 reported having given such advice: about half indicated that they had discussed sexual matters with their patient. (As previously noted, in nearly 90 percent of the cases, the physician was the same doctor who had treated the patient for his first heart attack one year previously, so the patient report cannot be explained away by the fact that the physicians had only recently begun treating the patient. Thus, there is some obvious discrepancy.) As to reports on *no advice* on sex relations having been provided, the range is from about 80 percent (by patient statement) to nearly 50 percent (by physician statement).

Among those few patients who reported receiving physician advice on sex (N=11), there was apparently sufficient coverage to fulfill their wishes for information. About 90 percent of this small group responded in the affirmative when asked if they felt they had received sufficient advice on the matter. This leaves, however, the remainder of that sub-group, which, in combination with the sizeable population remaining, either had been given no advice or received inadequate advice, according to their own report.

SUMMARY

In this chapter we have examined the reported use of various types of resources by patients. These were chiefly resources in the community: health and social service institutions and various types of professionals. After discharge from the hospital, there was one prominent and obvious resource with whom there was continued contact throughout the year: the physician. There was relatively low agency usage, aside from those services providing directly for medical needs. Although our data do not deal directly with the issue, in part this pattern may have been due to actual minimal need for services other than those of the physician. In part it may have been due to physician choices concerning need for referral. According to the data from patients, the clergy and cardiac rehabilitation clinics were little utilized as additional sources of support. The communication between physician and patient dealt with areas on which patients received and/or wanted advice. Some problems of communication between less educated patients and physicians were reported, primarily in the period shortly before discharge from the hospital (T_1).

NOTES

1. Twenty-seven percent of the patients were served by doctors who graduated from Tufts Medical School: 21 percent from Harvard Medical; 11 percent from Boston University; two other schools ranked next in proportion: 5.4 percent from Middlesex Medical School, and 5.1 percent from Columbia Medical School. The rest of the patients were treated by graduates of other Medical Schools.
2. See Chapter 2 for a detailed explanation of physician ratings of patient health status.
3. Chi-square = 14.55, df = 4, p < .01; gamma = −.32.
4. Use of services depends in part on (a) availability, (b) need, and (c) referral, among other factors. At this point, given the direction of our data, it is difficult to assess whether there were actual needs which might have been met but were not. One aspect of this situation is that, as will be seen, physicians made minimal referrals to agencies and other professionals. Whether this is because they perceived no need or because of their own lack of information on relevant resources remains problematic.

    In contrast to the data reported here, it appears that considerable proportions of patients made use of services of non-institutional resources, such as family, friends, and neighbors. This point and its implications are considered in some detail in Chapter 7.

5. The pages following draw upon materials appearing in Croog and Levine, 1969.
6. Chi-square = 15.18, df = 2, p < .001.
7. These areas are recorded in Table 4. On the whole, items could be classified easily within relevant categories. For example, if a patient expressed an interest in what food he should eat, or avoid eating, this interest would be coded as "diet." Similarly, one interested in how much weight he should lose, would have his concern coded as "weight."

   On the other hand, criteria for the following four areas deserve some explanation:

   Prognosis: This category reflected patient concern with his progress, when and if he might expect a recurrence of a heart attack, the course of the illness, and how long a period of convalescence he could expect.

   Work: "Work" reflected questions pertaining to the type of work the patient may do, the number of hours he may work, the date on which he may expect to return to work, etc.

   Therapy: In this category were placed general questions on how the patient might prevent further attacks, and how he ought to take care of himself.

   Activity: Coded under this category were responses dealing with matters of activities permissible and non-permissible. These primarily dealt with physical exertion and included questions on how often a patient may climb stairs, how much exercise he may take per day, whether he may drive a car, whether to watch television late at night, whether he may do odd jobs around the house, etc.
8. Distribution of the study population of 345 men in terms of the variables examined were as follows: (a) one year of college or more, 24.0 percent; four years of high school, 32.2 percent; three years of high school or less, 43.8 percent; (b) Hollingshead Index of Social Position, I (highest) 4.1 percent; II, 11.6 percent; III, 18.2 percent; IV, 44.1 percent; V, 22.0 percent; (c) patients with private physicians: 64.5 percent; "service" or "ward" patients: 35.5 percent; (d) age 30 through 39 years, 9.8 percent; 40 through 49 years, 36.0 percent; 50 through 60 years, 54.2 percent.
9. For a listing of the self-rating personality items, refer to Note 4-6, Chapter 1. For additional information see: Burgess and Wallin, 1953 and B. Farber, 1900.
10. The five additional items were the latter five listed in Reference 4-6 in Chapter 1. For discussion of their hypothetical relation to

the etiology of the illness, refer to: Friedman and Rosenman, 1974; C.D. Jenkins et al., 1971; C.D. Jenkins, 1971; D. Kenigsberg et al., 1974; S.L. Syme, 1975 and Wardwell and Bahnson, 1973.

11. All items in Table 5 on which patients reported advice had been covered by a specific question on each matter, with the exception of two. These exceptions were the items on sexual activity or future plans. At the conclusion of questions presented as a listing by the interviewer, patients were asked: "Was there anything else the doctor advised you about?" Those who mentioned sexual performance or some aspect of future plans were coded accordingly. Other items were mentioned so infrequently, i.e., by one or two patients out of 345, that they were not of sufficient dimension to be included in the table. These items pertained to such matters as symptoms and interpersonal relations.

12. These areas of advice are consistent with those commonly given by physicians to heart patients in a therapeutic and rehabilitative regimen. For example, see Friedman and Rosenman, 1974; Naughton and Hellerstein, 1973; and N.F. Wenger et al., 1970.

Chapter 6

PHYSICIAN ADVICE AND COMPLIANCE ORIENTATION

INTRODUCTION

In the previous chapter we reviewed briefly the pattern of advice from physicians as perceived by patients. The review was part of our effort to document the experience of the heart patients, in this case in relation to a key support figure in their "armory of resources" during the illness—the physician. We turn now to another aspect of the area of advice: the matter of disposition toward compliance with perceived physician advice.

COMPLIANCE ORIENTATION AND PATIENT REPORTING

Considering the advice which was given in regard to the various life areas, what was the pattern of reported compliance and positive intention? What variables were

191

related to differing levels of reported compliance in each of the areas?[1]

That compliance with physician advice is of critical importance in the care of heart patients is a widely accepted precept in medicine. In recent years it has received an increasing amount of discussion and analysis. The literature in this area ranges from hortatory accounts and philosophical statements to empirical studies of compliance with medical regimen and health education efforts (see, for example, Becker et al., 1972, 1974; Marston, 1970; Mitchell, 1974; Johannsen et al., 1966). Various theoretical models have been developed to help explain and predict patient compliance behavior, both in regard to specific illnesses and illness in general (Hochbaum, 1958; Kasl and Cobb, 1966; Kegeles, 1963, 1969; Kirscht, 1974; Rosenstock, 1960).

The problems of studying and measuring compliance are well known and need no extended rehearsal here. Some few examples can perhaps suffice. Unfortunately, there are few tools available for measuring conformity with advice which involves complex behavior, which must be carried out for a long period, and which is not easily susceptible to scrutiny. The problem of classification of level of actual compliance is a major one, particularly when one deals with areas of advice which are varied and of differing levels of specificity. Further, one can make no assumptions that compliance in one area is indicative of compliance in others; this is an empirical question on which adequate research is yet to be done. In brief, the whole area of compliance behavior is one in which major conceptual and methodological advances still remain to be made. Our approach here, therefore, is to proceed in a conservative manner in both reporting and interpreting our findings, presenting the data as part of our larger documentation of aspects of patient experience over the course of a year.

Compliance Behavior and Compliance Orientation: Some Key Distinctions

In an article some years ago Davis usefully pointed out that compliance behavior should be kept conceptually separate from compliant attitudes. As an attitude, he wrote, compliance consists of a willingness or orientation toward doing what the doctor advises. "In its behavioral aspect, however, compliance can be said to exist only when the patient actually carries out his doctor's orders" (Davis, 1968).

Our concern is with one key dimension of the attitude phenomenon: the "compliance orientation." This is operationally defined as the direction of expressed willingness of the patient to comply with an item of advice, as indicated by his report of compliance behavior. The responses are viewed for our analytic purposes as reflecting a compliance attitude or frame of mind—a willingness and intention to obey instructions of the physician.[2]

If patients responded at T_2 that they had received advice from their physicians in a particular area, they were also asked about their compliance concerning the item. They were asked, "How well have you been able to follow the doctor's advice?" on such matters as medications, diet, exercise, and the like. The responses were coded: "completely," "for the most part," "somewhat," "not at all." On some items dealing with areas of future behavior they were asked, "How well do you think you will be able to follow the doctor's advice?" For example, patients at home for one month would have to respond in terms of intent in regard to compliance with advice on part-time employment or changing work habits. Further, the replies on other items such as avoiding quarrels or reducing smoking, while dealing in part with the past, also linked into the future.

For initial analysis, the responses were coded in terms of three categories: complete compliance, partial compliance, and non-compliance. The middle category is composed of the two intermediate response groups, "for the most part" and "somewhat."

We further distinguished two types of compliance orientation frames: that of (a) positive complier and (b) non-complier. The positive complier is the patient who reports complete compliance with the advice. The negative one is the patient who reports that he will comply (1) not at all or (2) partially.

The inclusion of "partial compliance" in the non-compliance orientation category is based upon the rationale that reported partial compliance is more indicative of non-compliance than it is of intended or actual compliance. From the medical standpoint, the partial compliers may be seen as a problem group along with the non-compliers. For example, the patient who is given medications for treatment of his heart disease, then only "partially" complies, is one who clearly belongs in another care category than the patients who cooperate fully in taking their medicine.

The materials on compliance orientation are drawn from two points in time: the T_2 and the T_3 stages. Although the total study period was one year, we have selected the T_2 period for special examination for several reasons: it enables the scrutiny of materials pertinent to a clear-cut illness experience. Further, the period of recall of physician advice in regard to management after hospitalization is relatively short. If we had selected the T_3 period, this would have meant dealing with a set of heterogenous experiences and with advice relevant to differing kinds of situations. Some patients, for example, were rehospitalized at differing points in the year, others developed additional ailments, and still others remained free of symptoms and had limited contacts with their doctors. To explore compliance orientation in regard to particular situations or time periods over the year in such instances would run the risk of contamination of recollections because of multiple hospitalizations, experiences, and ailments, as well as the passage of time.

This focus on compliance orientation is, of course, quite different from a focus on actual patient behavior in regard to the areas of physician advice. Some additional indirect evidence is available, however, from other sources. These include assessment by the physicians as well as patient reports on such matters as change in smoking pattern and in physical exertion. The materials appear at a later point in the chapter.

Compliance Orientation and Medical Advice: Distributions at T_2

In Table 1 we present data on areas of reported physician advice and the responses of patients concerning compliance at T_2. On each item the table excludes the responses of those who had earlier indicated that they had received no advice in regard to the matter. The items are ordered according to the proportion of patients receiving the advice who also indicated compliance orientation as defined earlier.

These advice items, as listed in the table, differ greatly in terms of the demands required for fulfillment. There are many dimensions on which they can be differentiated. These include variations in specificity, length of time required, degree of judgment, degree of participation and of cooperation by other persons, and apparent immediacy or relevance of the item for recovery. For example, the advice on time of return to work involves fulfilling a specific recommendation by the physician at one particular time. The issue of weight control is very different, however, as it requires a series

Table 1. Advice From Physicians and Compliance Orientation of Patients at T_2.
Compliance Orientation of Those Patients Advised on Each Item.
Listed by Magnitude of "Complete" C-O Column Percentages Within Each Category

Advice Area	N Receiving Advice as Percent of Total Patient Population (345)		Patient Reported Compliance Orientation					
			Complete*		Partial*		Not at All*	
	N	Percent	N	Percent	N	Percent	N	Percent
Medical Regimen								
Medication	307	89.0	271	88.3	36	11.7	–	–
Diet	276	80.0	175	63.4	96	34.8	5	1.8
Weight	226	65.5	123	54.4	92	40.7	11	4.9
Reduction of Health Risks								
Alcohol Usage	174	50.4	137	78.7	33	19.0	4	2.3
Smoking	252	73.0	148	58.7	75	29.8	29	11.5
Exercise and Physical Straining								
Lifting Things	206	59.7	174	84.5	28	13.6	4	1.9
Exercise	135	39.1	102	75.6	28	20.7	5	3.7
Walking	274	79.4	196	71.5	71	25.9	7	2.6
Climbing Stairs	266	77.1	189	71.1	74	27.8	3	1.1
Resting	187	54.2	120	64.2	66	35.3	1	.5
Work Arrangements								
Time of Work Return	246	71.3	196	79.7	35	14.2	15	6.1
Part-time Work	176	51.0	123	69.9	25	14.2	28	15.9
Different Job-Same Place	51	14.8	31	60.8	3	5.9	17	33.3
Different Job-New Place	25	7.2	13	52.0	5	20.0	7	28.0
Emotional Stress								
Avoiding Quarrels, Upsetting Events	148	42.9	63	42.6	76	51.3	9	6.1
Agencies								
Agencies-Financial Help	8	2.3	8	100.0	–	–	–	–
Agencies-Medical Care	5	1.4	3	60.0	2	40.0	–	–
Agencies-Rehabilitation	4	1.2	1	25.0	–	–	3	75.0
Other								
Recreation Activities	60	17.4	53	88.3	5	8.3	2	3.4
Vacations	21	6.1	15	71.4	5	23.8	1	4.8
Change in Living Arrangements (Home)	26	7.5	17	65.4	4	15.4	5	19.2

* Phrasing refers to actual patient response concerning degree of compliance
with medical advice. See text for discussion of compliance orientation
and wording of questions.

of repeated decisions by the individual, changes in life style, participation and cooperation by others, willingness to undergo deprivation, and performance of the restrictive behavior into the indefinite future. Further, the acts of violation of restriction are not immediately relevant. Eating a chocolate sundae or an eclair is not seen as a prelude to a heart attack. The effects are believed to be distant and they can easily be rationalized away.

As the table shows, substantial proportions of those advised described themselves as positive compliers on some individual items. In terms of interview response at least, these materials reflect resolution and interest at this particular point in following recommendations presented by the physician, the key authority figure in the therapy.

It is difficult to find a clear pattern of positive compliance in percentages according to type of advice given and the varied dimensions listed above. For example, while items dealing with specific instructions, such as medications and time of work return rank high, so also do those which deal with more general precepts, such as that the patient should arrange for more recreational activities. The ranking itself, however, may indicate which particular areas of conformance were seen by patients as being the more difficult. These include weight control, smoking, and changing jobs. For a middle-aged man to change his job and his place of employment, for example, may constitute a profound change in his life, associations, and income potential, and it is clearly easier to consider than it is to achieve. Further, the general precept to avoid quarrels and upsetting situations is not one which can be simply attained by the energies and intent of the individual alone.

Another way of approaching compliance orientation and its role in the total experience of the heart patient is to examine the frequencies of responses other than complete compliance. These perhaps should first be considered in terms of their meaning in the context of the interview. It would be easy for patients, after reviewing the advice received, to indicate to the interviewer that they were following it. Such an approach bears no penalties and in fact may be the easier course, indicating that the patients are, after all, sensible men willing to follow the authority of the physician. Saying they would comply completely entails no obligation to do so, and patients were well aware that they could follow their own course no matter what they verbalized. Obviously, among those who maintain they would not comply at all—or who would do so only partially—the probability of repeated compliance behavior over time is less likely than among men who claimed to be "complete compliers" (Kegeles, 1967).

As the table shows, on numerous items from one-fourth to one-half the men advised indicated that they would do other than follow the doctor's advice completely. On even a matter of clear medical relevance, the taking of medications, about one man in ten at T_2 indicated that he would not follow the regimen set up by the doctor. Hence, it is not surprising that on other matters pertaining to life style, work, and the visceral pleasures considerably more patients indirectly indicated resistance to following the doctor's advice. Relatively large percentages, for example, were expressing doubt about changing jobs, about undertaking part-time work, and making changes in their living arrangements. In fact, as the third column shows, on some items one-fifth to one-third of those advised directly stated complete non-compliance orientations.

One way of evaluating the meaning of compliance and non-compliance orientations is to look at the life pattern of each man and to evaluate the significance of the item of advice in his life. For example, among the men who were advised to change their living arrangements in the home, their compliance could be evaluated in terms of feasibility. The man living in a crowded apartment in a fourth-floor walk-up tenement and who cannot comply with restrictions on walking stairs is in an obviously different category from the person who owns his own spacious home. The meaning of non-compliance in regard to the weight and diet items might be evaluated in terms of cultural traditions, ethnic origins, class level, standards of body image in the immediate social group, the meaning of food, modes of dealing with anxiety through oral means, etc. Thus, one may hypothesize that the products in each of the compliance categories may be the end result of a set of heterogeneous factors, rather than a single dimension. As noted earlier, however, there is a literature rich in hypotheses in regard to factors related to differential patterns of compliance with advice and factors underlying social influence, leadership, and subjection to authority. In the next section we consider some of these lines of explanation and review some attempts at exploring relationships in the heart patient data.

Variables Related to Compliance Orientation

How can the differences in degree of reported compliance orientation be explained? As the literature in this area points out, there are a great number of factors which bear on the problem, including many of a social, psychological, structural, and process nature.[3] In an effort to explore the possible correlates of reported compliance orientation, a series of variables were selected to be cross-tabulated against each item individually. These were drawn from several principal dimensions on which we had collected data from patients. They were

(1) social and personal characteristics: age, occupation, educational level, (2) psychological self-rating traits, as indicated by a series of items on which patients were asked to rate themselves, and (3) perceived subjective health level as indicated by number of symptoms reported.[4]

To carry out this effort, a series of compliance items were drawn from the larger list of advice areas covered by physicians, in order that sufficient numbers would be present in cells for tests of association using non-parametric techniques. (See Table 5, Chapter 5 for the complete listing.) These items, while selected in part on the basis of numbers receiving advice, also reflect principal areas of advice. Thus, they include:

1. *Medical Regimen*
    A. Taking medications
    B. Dietary restrictions (as low cholesterol diet, etc.)
    C. Weight control
2. *Reduction of Health Risks*
    D. Smoking reduction
    E. Alcohol usage
3. *Exercise and Physical Straining*
    F. Exercise
    G. Lifting
    H. Rest
4. *Work Arrangements*
    I. Date of return to work
    J. Working part-time
5. *Emotional Stress*
    K. Avoiding quarrels and emotionally upsetting events.

As indicated in Chapter 1, these procedures were informed by a series of underlying hypotheses: (a) that level of reported compliance orientation is associated with age, (b) that level of reported compliance orientation varies by social status level, as indicated by educational level, and (c) that level of reported compliance orientation varies by personality trait. These hypotheses in turn are based on research findings as well as clinical experience of physicians. These findings show, for example, that less compliance is found among persons of lower social status, that men with particular personality characteristics are more amenable to authority and more likely to comply, and that age is a significant variable in affecting health-related behavior (Becker and Maiman, 1975; Davis and Eichhorn, 1963; Marston, 1970; Vincent, 1971).

The results of the analysis, however, produced few significant associations. Education, for example, was not associated with a single one of the advice-compliance items. On one item, smoking, there was a significant association between occupational level and expressed compliance: the higher the status, the greater the compliance orientation.[5] Age was associated with willingness to conform to dietary advice:[6] there was a significant difference between men under 40 and those above that age, with the older men indicating higher compliance. Some significant relationships emerged from a series of personality self-rating items, although there was no broad consistent patterning. The associations were as follows: self-characterization of "eating rapidly" was negatively associated with a compliance in weight control and with avoiding quarrels or upsetting events. Being in a hurry was negatively associated with willingness to comply in working part-time.[7] Being nervous or irritable and "easily depressed" were each positively associated with compliance in taking medications.

Since such a large number of cross-tabulations were run, it is inevitable that some of the significant results could have emerged purely through chance. The fact

that so few variables were related to compliance orientation may be a product of the types of measures used,
their relative sensitivity or their validity. Consistent failure to discover strong positive findings in regard to
social variables, however, may be significant in pointing
toward more subtle variables and complex underlying
processes in this illness.

Compliance Orientation: An Appraisal of Patterning

Thus far we have examined compliance orientation in
relation to individual items of advice, and the focus has
been upon the nature of the advice item itself. We now
turn to consider these data at another level. In this study
population of heart patients, the number of items of
advice provided to individuals by physicians varied considerably. In responding to each item, individual patients
indicated that on some items they were complying, but
on others they were not. Our first purpose here, therefore, is to describe the pattern of compliance orientation.

A second question concerns compliance orientation
in relation to number of items of advice given. Some
researchers have reported that when patients receive
advice on many issues, they are less likely to
comply than those who receive advice on only a few issues. In the case of the heart patients, we report on this
issue of non-compliance because of "overload."

Another problem for review concerns the correlates
of the compliance orientation, when considered as a
dimension in itself. Patients can be characterized by
degree of reported compliance on a series of items. Do
low, medium, and high compliers vary in terms of personal, social or psychological dimensions? Are there useful predictor variables which can identify patients in
advance in terms of their likely compliance orientation?
This is our third area for exploration here.

The Compliance Orientation Index (C-O Index)

In order to examine compliance orientation as a syndrome of responses to a series of items, an index was employed based on the selected 11 individual response items cited earlier.[8] A Compliance Orientation Index (or C-O Index) was calculated according to the following formula:

$$\frac{B \times 100}{A} = \text{compliance orientation percentage}$$

where A = number of items of advice reported by the patient

and B = number of items of complete compliance reported by the patient

For the purposes of analysis, it should be noted that only the responses indicating complete compliance are included in the Index. We assume that this response, whether followed through consistently or not, reflects a clear-cut positive statement of an attitude of cooperation with the physician. At the same time, for our purposes here, we assume that a statement of "partial response" indicates sufficient negative aspects to warrant its not being classified as reflecting a "positive compliance" frame of mind.

In Table 2 we report the percentage distributions deriving from the C-O Index. As may be seen, the proportion indicating positive compliance orientation toward 80 percent of the advice items amounted to 42 percent of the total population. At the other end of the range, the percentage who would comply completely with less than 50 percent of the advice given amounted to only 15 percent. Thus, in terms of the expressed compliance responses in the interviews, this population was highly oriented toward positive compliance.

Turning now to the issue of compliance attitude and information overload, we can consider the relationship

Table 2. Score on Compliance Orientation Index.
Distribution of Total Population.
At T_2. N = 344.

Compliance Orientation Index Score*	Number of Patients	Percent of Total Study Population	Cumulative Percent
0	6	1.7	1.7
1-19	11	3.2	4.9
20-29	11	3.2	8.1
30-39	14	4.1	12.2
40-49	11	3.2	15.4
50-59	45	13.1	28.5
60-69	42	12.2	40.7
70-79	59	17.2	57.9
80-89	69	20.0	77.9
90-99	5	1.5	79.4
100	71	20.6	100.0
Total	344**	100.0	

* Score indicates the proportion of areas of advice given to which the patient has indicated full compliance orientation. For example, 17 patients have scores indicating compliance with 19 percent or less of the advice items which they were given by their physicians. See text.

** N = 344 rather than 345 since one patient reported receiving no advice at T_2.

between expressed compliance orientation and number of items reported. The study population was divided into three groups in terms of the proportions of scores on the C-O Index. Those with a score of 59 percent and under were termed "low" while those with scores of from 80 to 100 percent were designated "high." The intermediate sector, ranging from 60 to 79 percent on the Index, was designated the "medium" group. The initial effort for trichotomization was to obtain three groups relatively equal in size. The skewed nature of the distribution led to some difficulty in doing this. The final grouping as a percentage of the total study population was as follows: low—28 percent; medium—29 percent; and high—42 percent.

Percentages were examined, comparing each of the three groups on compliance score according to number of items of advice received. Numbers of items of advice were combined, particularly for the lower levels, in order to have sufficient numbers for reasonable report on percentages. No relationship was found between number of items of advice and scores for the C-O Index.

What is the meaning of this finding? In terms of expressed orientation toward compliance, the number of items which a physician advises on does not appear to make much difference. The expressed willingness of patients to comply, according to these data, is not a function of number of items reported, and the simplistic hypothesis of "information overload" is not supported. With this finding in mind, we turn to a related task, the exploration of possible relevance of *other* variables to differential scores on the C-O Index.

Compliance Orientation Index: An Exploration of Correlates at T_2

What are the social and psychological variables which are related to compliance orientations and which may be used as possible predictors of scores on the C-O Index?[9] Following our usual procedures, a series of cross tabulations were carried out in order that possible relationships with some selected variables might be scrutinized. No significant relationships were found which merit reporting here.

The meaning of this lack of significant statistical results deserves only conservative assessment. Viewed in a positive sense, the results show that expressed compliance orientation is influenced by "a different drummer" than the phenomena represented by the variables reviewed here. In the case of an illness as serious as this, with its threat of possible immediate and unpredictable death, the facts of the illness itself may lead to a particular compliance orientation. If one is to live, there are certain rules and restrictions which must be obeyed. The impact of these rules, their meaning, and the authority of the physician who transmits them may override the possible influences of social status variables, cultural beliefs, and personality traits. In this case, the issue may be viewed at T_2 as a clear life-and-death matter—one so clear in its dimension that there are few alternate choices for patients.

At the same time, it must be noted that other elements can be cited to account for the results shown here: the character of the indices, the nature of response in the interview situation, response set, the possibility that the really influential variables were not tested, as well as other factors. Clearly the issue deserves further testing with more sophisticated methods and instruments and concepts. The ostensible lack of relationship may be itself a meaningful statement of relationship, indicating some important data about the powerful influence of life threat in inducing compliance.

Compliance Orientation at T_3

At the end of the study year, despite the heterogeneous health experience of the men following the first hospitalization, most patients were still expected to be following advice from their physician in regard to their health. When asked a series of questions about the advice they were currently supposed to be following, 97 percent mentioned at least one item. About three-fourths

(77 percent) mentioned four or more areas on which they were currently supposed to be following advice of the physician. Thus, after one year nearly all the men surveyed in the study who previously had no major illness in their lives, were now perceiving themselves as still subject to some elements of the medical regimen.

This point, while simple to phrase, tells a great deal about the transformation of the lives of the patients over the course of the year. From men who had had a lifetime free from significant illness, they were now living with the new perception of themselves: as persons whose current and future health depended in part on changes in life patterns and personal habits.

The pattern of expressed compliance orientation at the end of the year is similar in many respects to that at T_2. In the final interview patients were asked questions similar to those at T_2, except that 10 principal areas were covered, rather than the longer listing. Then, as at the earlier instance, they were asked about the degree to which they were complying, except that the question dealt with current performance.

As may be seen in Table 3, two-thirds to three-quarters of the total study population reported that they were supposed to be following advice on such matters as weight control, exercise, diet, smoking, taking medications, and their work.

Comparison with Table 1 indicates that the general picture of advice to be followed at one year is similar to that for the period one month subsequent to discharge from the hospital. At one year, therefore, for these proportions, the burden of their heart ailment remains with them in the sense of requiring that they take care in key areas of their lives and in their personal habits. The requirements, of course, were not as strict for all these men as they were at T_1.

Direct comparison between items in Table 1 and

Table 3. Areas of Advice Given and Positive Compliance Orientation at T_3.
Master List at T_3. N = 293.

Advice Area	Percent of Total Reporting Advice From Physicians	Of Those Advised, Percent With Positive Compliance Orientation
1. Exercise	74.1	51.6
2. Weight Reduction	74.1	42.3
3. Medications	66.3	90.2
4. Food Habits, Special Diets	65.0	48.8
5. Smoking	65.0	44.2
6. Work	64.6	59.2
7. Resting	49.5	55.2
8. Avoiding Quarrels	40.4	22.8
9. Drinking	36.6	63.5
10. Sexual Activity	18.2	56.6

Table 3 cannot be made, since the nature of advice varied from T_2 to T_3. For example, advice about work at T_2 centered in large degree on date of return to work or on such matters as changing type of employment or switching to a part-time job. At T_3, given the heterogeneous health picture of the study population, the specific nature of work advice varied. Nevertheless, on a small series of items some light comparison can be made, insofar as the character of the advice remained essentially the same at T_2 and T_3.

Among those patients who had been given a regimen for taking medications, 89 percent at T_2 and 90 percent at T_3 indicated positive compliance orientation. On the matter of advice on food habits or special diets, 63 percent at T_2 65 percent at T_3 reported positive compliance orientation. On other items which could be compared there was a drop of between 10 and 20 percent between the two stages among those who were given advice and who were participants in both stages. These are as follows in terms of percentages, first at T_2, then at T_3: weight reduction, 54 percent versus 42 percent; advice on smoking, 58 versus 44; alcohol usage, 78 versus 64, and avoiding quarrels, 42 versus 23. Thus, on these items, the relative ranking remained similar from T_2 to T_3, with a decline in positive compliance orientation. In this listing, as well as in the larger series in the tables from which they were drawn, substantial proportions were not indicating a positive compliance orienta tion. If we assume that positive intentions to comply do not necessarily lead to compliance, then it would appear that there may well be even less compliance among those who are ambivalent or who express outright negative attitudes.

The items on quarrels and sex deserve special note, since one deals with an ambiguous instruction and the other with a relatively sensitive issue. About the same proportion of men at T_2 and T_3 reported advice from the physician on avoiding quarrels and upsetting events. Thus, in terms of proportions at least, there was high continuity in level of the total population who were to avoid interpersonal stresses. At the end of the year, however, the proportion of men with a positive compliance orientation in this matter had declined to about one-fifth of those advised.

On the matter of sex, as we reported previously, a set of direct questions was asked at the third interview. Though only a minority of men reported advice, there was apparent high positive compliance orientation, similar to that for other items.

Compliance Orientation Index: The Case at One Year

Thus far we have been concerned with responses on

individual items as they reflect compliance orientation at T_3. As in the case of the data at T_2, it is also desirable to look beyond the individual items to the constellations of items as they were perceived and reported by patients. This procedure enables us to examine, at least in a modest way, the patterning of compliance orientation in more natural terms—since patients were given sets of items, and their responses are made to the sets as well as to the separate instructions.

The same procedure was followed at T_3 in regard to items on which patients reported they had received advice. In this case, the number of items examined was 10 rather than the 11 selected from the larger group for the T_2 phase. Hence, strict comparison is not possible. The percentages indicate in a general sense the relative response of patients to a series of items.

It will be recalled that for purposes of earlier analysis, the compliance responses were divided into three groups relatively similar in size, and these were labeled for differentiation. Using the same criteria at T_3 for comparison, the following results emerged: those patients at T_3 who were in the low positive orientation group (scoring from 0 to 59) constituted twice the percentage than found earlier (57 percent as compared with the 28.5 percent at T_2). At the other end of the range, the high group, the percentage drop reflects the increase at the low score end. From 42.2 percent at T_2 to 21 percent of the patients at T_3 had high scores (positive compliance orientation on 80 to 100 percent of items on which they were advised). For the medium score group (positive C-O on 60 to 79 percent of the items) the percentages were 17.6 at T_3 as compared with 31.3 at T_2.

The populations at both stages, it should be emphasized, are not precisely the same. The reduction from the initial 345 men to 293 respondents was due to losses from death and from those who refused to be interviewed. Thus, as noted above, one cannot automatically generalize from one to the other. In a paired comparison analysis, we selected for examination only those patients who responded at both T_2 and T_3. We charted whether their T_3 C-O score was higher, lower, or the same. The results for individual patients show the same patterning, consistent with the examination of C-O scores for the two total populations. For 18 percent of the patients, the C-O score was higher at T_3, indicating an expression of more positive compliance orientation than earlier. However, for 64 percent, the compliance orientation index was lower. For 17 percent, the C-O index remained the same as at T_2. The remaining group of ten men (3 percent) was a residual category, since they reported at T_3 that there was no advice from physicians which they should currently be following.

The reasons for these findings are not clear, and many explanations might be offered. At one year after the heart attack a considerable proportion of men were symptom-free and had not been rehospitalized during the year. Hence, it might be conjectured that their feelings of urgency in regard to compliance were reduced by return to health and normal life. This would mean, however, that one would expect to find positive compliance orientation among those men who had reported further difficulties during the year, who were rehospitalized, or who had developed additional symptoms of significant illness.

To test out this thesis, change in C-O scores in two stages was examined, comparing men most seriously ill over the year with those who had been relatively free of additional illness. The groups "rehospitalized" and "not rehospitalized but with significant symptoms" were compared with the patients classified as nonrehospitalized and without significant symptoms.[10] Two types of cross-tabulations were examined (N=293). One was designed to determine if "rehospitalization and symptoms" (i.e., higher severity of illness over the year) and compliance orientation level were related. No statistical association was found.

Next, three sub-groups were examined: those who changed upward in C-O Index score, those who remained at the same level, and those whose C-O score declined over the course of the year. Again, no statistically significant differences were found. These data imply that for this population at least, the apparent level of severity of illness during the study year was not related to level of reported compliance orientation. The hypothesis that the "sickest" people in the study population would tend to comply more was not borne out.

Level of Compliance: Physician Assessment and the Case of Smoking

As indicated earlier in this chapter, it is not possible to present data here in regard to the complex issues of the relationships between compliance orientation and actual compliance behavior. As part of our effort to document the experience of the study population, however, it may be useful to review physician assessment and changes in smoking pattern. These may serve to indicate at least in a general sense the possible direction of patient performance.

In a questionnaire completed by 269 physicians at the end of the study year, questions were asked concerning their assessment of patient compliance in some of the chief areas on which advice had been given. Fixed alternative responses were "good," "fair," and "poor." Among those men who had been given advice on each item, physicians reported on compliance according to the following distributions:

	Good	Fair	Poor	Total Percent
Activity restriction	73.2	21.3	5.5	100.0
Limitation on responsibility	69.9	18.1	12.0	100.0
Advice on diet	62.7	22.1	15.2	100.0
Regular physical exercise	67.2	23.3	9.4	100.0
Smoking restriction	69.3	15.1	15.6	100.0

Assessing those patients whom they had advised, the physicians apparently had a generally positive impression of performance. The majority of patients were seen as complying in some degree ("good" or "fair"). Moreover, the major segment of these, as indicated in the data above, were seen as "good" compliers. These results are congruent with the findings of other investigators (Kasl, 1975) which have indicated that physicians tend to over-estimate the amount of patient compliance. We have no way of knowing how familiar each physician was with the actual compliance of patients in each of the areas. These assessments are themselves a component of the interaction system between patient and physician, however. They constitute one basis by which physicians make further decisions in regard to the therapeutic regimen, the progress of the patient, and the need for further medical intervention.

Regardless of whether the "poor" compliance category is considered too large or too small, it is apparent that the *physician* view of patients appraises the trend of compliance in a way similar to that shown by patient compliance orientation. The direction they perceive is toward complying or making efforts toward compliance. In this illness situation, few among physicians or patients give indications other than that lives have changed and that changes must be made to facilitate health and survival.

The individual ratings by physicians were further classified into a crude index of assessed compliance for individual patients. On the basis of physician ratings for each of these items, a classification was made. Score 1 was given if the physician rated the patient's compliance as "good" on all items on which he reported advice. If the ratings were mixed, including mainly "good" or "fair," a score of 2 was given. Mixed ratings, including mostly "fair" or "poor" compliance, received a rating of 3. The final category was one in which all ratings of compliance were "poor." A residual category was reserved for those cases in which the physician made no assessment of compliance. In the total population for which ratings were given (N=269) the score distribution was as follows:

Score	Percent
1	43.9
2	39.8
3	4.8
4	4.1
No Rating	7.4

Thus, it would appear that the physicians themselves are heavily inclined toward rating favorably the compliance performance of their patients, with nearly four-fifths reported to be in the upper categories.

This index and the individual ratings, as we have noted, serve as crude indicators of physician beliefs concerning how well their patients are performing. Since they are crude assessments, we have chosen not to deal in detail with the ratings or to examine their correlates. The ratings were made on the basis of clinician judgment and the parameters for decision were not specified in the interview instructions. Nor do we have information to permit evaluation of the accuracy and adequacy of the ratings themselves. They serve here, however, as part of the emerging picture of doctor patient relations, as it appears in this history of the heart patient during the study year.

Added to the complexity of assessment of compliance is the fact that the patient may comply not because of the doctor, but for other reasons. Much of the advice given by individual physicians is also affirmed and imparted from other sources. Thus, restrictions on heavy drinking or excessive weight are common precepts in social groups, and the fact that a person drinks moderately or tries to keep a trim figure may be the result of diverse social influences. Nevertheless, it may be useful here to review briefly the data in a key area of advice which is commonly given to heart patients: smoking reduction or elimination. Here it is possible to compare responses by the patient at two points in time, as well as assessment by the physician of his performance.

Illness, Advice and Change: The Case of Smoking

In the interview at T_2 patients were asked questions concerning use of cigarettes, pipes, cigars, etc., in the period before the heart attack.[11] For purposes of examining change, we shall deal with cigarette smoking only. Judging by their own responses, the patient population was characterized by relatively high use of cigarettes in the pre-illness period. (See Table 4.) The general level of smoking in the total patient population was relatively high—as many as 42 percent smoked two packs or more per day. Nineteen percent were nonsmokers.

These data may be compared with information from other studies of the smoking practices of males carried out around the time of the interview program. For example, a study by Hammond and Garfinkel (Hammond and Garfinkel, 1961, 1963) reports the following

Table 4.   Cigarette Smoking Level at Three Stages:
Before Hospitalization, T_2, and T_3.

Cigarettes Per Day	Prior To Hospitalization N = 345	T_2 N = 345	T_3 N = 293
None	19.4	69.8	58.4
1- 9	2.6	8.3	7.1
10	1.4	5.0	6.9
11-19	2.7	2.9	4.4
20	19.1	7.6	11.3
21-39	13.1	2.6	5.8
40-59	31.0	3.5	5.7
60 or more	10.7	.3	.4
Total Percentage	100.0	100.0	100.0

percentages in cigarette consumption among men in the modal age group for this study, 50-60: a) none or occasional cigarettes, 50 percent; b) 1 to 9 cigarettes, 5 percent; c) 10 to 19 cigarettes, 9 percent; d) 20 cigarettes, 18 percent; e) 21 to 39 cigarettes, 10 percent; and f) 40 or more cigarettes, 6.5 percent. The data are based on a national study. Similar rates have been reported in other studies as well (Shapiro et al., 1969).

In the Hammond-Garfinkel group those smoking two packs or more per day amounted to 6.5 percent of the total, whereas 6 to 7 times as many men in our study (42 percent) smoked that heavily.

Thus, by these and other comparisons, it appears that the study population constituted a group highly devoted to the use of cigarettes in the period before the heart attack. These data, while perhaps conforming to current hypotheses concerning the role of cigarette smoking in heart disease, should not be construed as any evidence for the thesis of cigarette smoking in etiology. That is another issue. They are presented here solely to set on record the nature of the distribution of cigarette smoking in this population, showing that tobacco use was not inconsiderable.

By the end of the year marked change in cigarette use had occurred. The number of non-smokers had increased markedly from the initial 19 percent to 58 percent. The number of cigarettes consumed by the continuing smokers had dropped markedly. Only six percent of the total were now in the two pack or more per day category. This group constituted 15 percent of the total still smoking. It is interesting to note that these post-illness figures are close to the distribution reported by Hammond and Garfinkel.

One feature of this phenomenon is that virtually all the smokers reported that they had been advised by their physicians concerning their tobacco consumption.[12] It would be naive to assume that this marked reduction was due only to physician influence—that men stopped smoking or reduced simply because their physicians told them to do so. Change in behavior of this type is the product of multiple influences, including personal decision, the weight of authority from multiple sources, such as those from the Heart Association, advertising, newspaper and magazine articles and influence of family members. At the same time, however, it may be important not to overlook the significance of physician advice in this area. Whether or not it is the sole factor, physician advice in a situation of ambiguity and uncertainty provided some specific steps to take, and these in turn were well supported by multiple sources of information and by a body of evidence based on scientific authority.

Among the patients who had stopped smoking, the reason most frequently cited was the advice of the physician. When asked an open-ended question about why they had stopped, 51 percent mentioned physician advice. The next major item cited was the patient's report that he decided to do so for health reasons. Thus, though the patient described himself as deciding the matter, it is difficult to disentangle this from the influence of the physician, as well as from other sources of information and advice. Further, the timing is of interest here. Virtually all of those who had given up smoking reported that they had done so early, by a week after discharge from hospital.

These data on reduction or stopping use of cigarettes are similar in some respects to that in other reports (Burt et al., 1974; Hay and Turbott, 1970; Werko, 1971; and Weinblatt et al., 1971). In the Hammond-Garfinkel study noted earlier, a population of men was reinterviewed after a two-year interval. Reduction or stopping was higher among those who reported having been hospitalized, and it was even higher among those who indicated that in the preceding period they had had heart disease, stroke, or high blood pressure. The authors conclude that "From this evidence it may be inferred that state of health has an influence on smoking habits" (Hammond and Garfinkel, 1963).

SUMMARY

In this chapter, we examined patient compliance orientation patterns in relation to physician advice. Reported compliance orientation was high for most items at T_2. Patients seemed to indicate less willingness to comply with advice dealing with more difficult or disruptive behavioral changes, such as weight control and changing jobs, however, possibly illuminating an area for therapeutic concern. One primary finding was that level of compliance orientation was generally unrelated to social and personal characteristics, psychological self-rating traits, number of symptoms reported, total number of items of advice received, and patient rehospitalization during the year. This lack of association could point either to the existence of more subtle variables or could serve to emphasize the powerful influence of the illness itself in inducing compliance.

Data at T_3 show a substantial decrease in positive compliance orientation as compared with the level following discharge from the hospital. This drop was not significantly related to the severity of illness or to the rehospitalization of the patient during the year.

Although compliance orientation, or patient willingness to comply, was the main emphasis of the chapter, attempts were also made to measure actual compliance behavior through the analysis of physician assessment of patient compliance performance and through a detailed examination of patient responses regarding smoking habits before and after the illness. Most physicians rated favorably the compliance performance of their patients, thus supporting the view of the patients themselves. This finding has some additional interest, since the physician's view of a patient's compliance often determines the direction of subsequent decisions and advice regarding the patient's medical regimen.

A comparison of patient descriptions of their smoking habits at two points in time permits a rough estimate of their actual compliance with physician's advice concerning smoking reduction. These data also supported the general trend of positive compliance which has already been noted. Patients reported that, prior to illness, 19 percent were nonsmokers and 42 percent smoked two or more packs per day. Thus the group fell into the category of relatively heavy smokers, according to national studies. At the end of the year, however, 58 percent reported themselves to be nonsmokers, and only six percent stated that they smoked two or more packs per day. The most frequently given reason for cessation of smoking was physician advice.

The relatively high level of compliance orientation, as seen from both patient and physician evidence, stands in contrast with reports of low compliance in the case of other illnesses. Multiple explanations have been suggested to account for these behavioral changes, including physician authority, personal decision, opinions of significant others, persuasive effects of the media, and response to the life threatening nature of heart disease.

NOTES

1. Although the term "adherence" is coming into more popular usage among professionals to describe the phenomenon reviewed here, we have chosen to employ the more commonly used term "compliance." The latter word has several meanings, as the dictionary tells us. The usage here is explicitly as follows: "to act in accordance with wishes, requests, commands, requirements, conditions, etc." No pejorative meaning is intended as far as this discussion of compliance with the medical regimen is concerned. Hence there seems little need to deal with other problems of meaning, such as reference to the term "adherence" might introduce.

2. In regard to the relationship between favorable orientation toward compliance and actual performance, Kegeles reports data from a study of motivation for obtaining examinations for cervical cancer. Although not a perfect predictor, the best indicator of subsequent follow-through in obtaining a cytological examination was stated intention to do so. Those persons who stated negative or ambivalent intentions usually did not obtain the examination. For additional information, see Kegeles, 1967.

3. As the literature in this area points out, there are a number of variables which might possibly bear on the problem. These include:

   1. Characteristics of the advice item itself (specificity, difficulty,

221

deprivation involved, costs, temporal nature, etc.)

2. Characteristics of the communicator, i.e., the physician (professional background, training, social characteristics, psychological traits, position in status systems, as those of the medical profession, hospital, community social structure, etc.)

3. Characteristics of the recipient (patient) and potential complier (social characteristics, psychological traits, position in status systems, nature of illness suffered, view of illness, experience in medical sphere (pre-programming), attitudinal systems, such as view of authority, comparative importance of health, etc.)

4. Characteristics of communication and communication process. Mode of delivery, timing, emotional tone, structure, and content of interaction system between doctor and patient.

5. Social structural elements and content of social setting. Elements in environment affecting compliance, as group norms, family norms, work situation, etc.

4. For a description of the measurement methods for these and other selected variables, refer to Note 4, Chapter 1.

5. Chi-square = 17.35, df = 4, p < .002; gamma = .33.

6. Chi-square = 12.58, df = 2, p < .002; gamma = .30.

7. This finding is consistent with hypotheses concerning "Type A" personality. See discussion and references in Chapter 8.

8. Index is similar to that employed by Davis, 1967.

9. To carry out these procedures, the trichotomized classification of the scores on the C-O Index was employed. (See text above for definition of grouping scores of High, Medium, Low.) These scores were then examined in relation to the following, some of which were used earlier in the analysis of individual items. These were: age, occupation, educational level, self-ratings on personality traits. In addition the following were also examined: (1) number of symptoms reported as current, (2) view on progress of the illness, (3) whether setbacks had been experienced, (4) belief that more might have been done by the physician to promote recovery, (5) feelings of uncertainty about the future. An index of marital disagreement was examined in relation to the compliance index. Finally, we explored the relationship to compliance orientation of variables indicating degree of experience with physicians and use of a regular physician previous to the heart attack.

10. See Chapter 2 for description of the categories and the criteria for classification.

11. For studies describing compliance with advice on smoking, refer to Davis and Eichhorn, 1963 and Davis, 1967.

12. This information is reflected in the responses of physicians to the mail questionnaire which they completed at Stage 2 (T_2). Virtually all physicians who had patients who smoked indicated they gave advice on cessation or reduction of cigarette use.

Chapter 7

THE PATIENT AND THE FAMILY:
LIFE WITH ILLNESS

INTRODUCTION

With this chapter we turn to consideration of the family of the patient, one of the most important elements in the "armory of resources." In the next pages we present data on the family through two perspectives: (a) the influence of the illness upon various aspects of family life and the lives of individual members and (b) the role of the family and of individual family members as supports, protective agents, and as sources of assistance. Each of these perspectives is given separate attention, although they overlap in many ways. For example, how the illness influences members of the family may affect in turn how they respond to the patient, and their interaction with him may influence the way in which he handles his illness and adjusts to his new situation as heart patient. In turn, this adjustment influences family members, and the cycle continues.

FAMILY MEMBERS AND LIFE CHANGES

Changes in Family Roles

The introduction of serious illness into a family may sometimes have pervasive effects upon the system of relationships among members. In the case of a heart attack in a parent, realignments and adjustments must be made to compensate for the incapacities which the illness brings to him. The processes are continuing ones, and the picture of realignments and role adaptations appears in different perspective, depending on the point in time at which it is observed. The first days after the heart attack, the picture at a month after hospitalization, and the progressive adaptations of roles over the course of succeeding months, all have their own unique features. Yet these role changes are extremely difficult to measure and assess, concerned as they are with changes at many levels. They involve changes in overt behavior, in emotional status, and in subtle nuances of interpersonal relations.

In this section we describe some aspects of the impact of illness upon the family. These include changes in the role of the patient, the wife, and the children. The materials here deal with a select subpopulation—those patients who were married at the time of first hospitalization. Reference to the small segment of unmarried, divorced, and widowed is omitted, insofar as small numbers preclude parallel analysis of the illness and their differing family arrangements.

One general feature of the role performance of the patient population is that at the end of the study year their level of activity in all spheres of life was less than it had been prior to the illness. According to their own self-assessment at T_3, 73 percent describe themselves as "less active" than they had been before the illness.

Further, although this was a trend among all patients, it was most pronounced among those who had been rated by their physicians as having made only a "partial" or "limited" recovery.[1]

Two variables point up more specific differences in the role of the man within the household: (a) the *amount* of activity of patients in doing "work around the house or apartment (as in painting, repairing, or other work like this)" and (b) *changes* in amount of activity in doing household chores. On the first item, there is a relationship in the direction of significance between physician rating and doing work around the house or apartment. at T_3, higher percentages of men rated as limited or partial in recovery rating (62 percent and 57 percent) reported that now they never did any work around the house, as compared with 41 percent of those with "full" recovery status who gave the same response. The higher the physician rating, the more likely the patient was to respond at T_3 "frequently" or "sometimes" in describing how often he worked around the house.

The relationship between health level and household activities is brought out more clearly in the second item. Here, respondents were asked to compare the amount of help they gave with household chores at two stages: (a) at T_3 and (b) before the occurrence of the heart attack. As may be seen in Table 1, about half of those in the partial and limited category and about one-third of those in the full recovery category reported they were doing less in the home. Relatively few in any category reported that they were doing more.

In evaluating these materials, it is important to note that the question concerning work around the house and household chores is itself social class-oriented. The question implies that all men are engaged in this type of activity, but obviously there are some to whom the question is minimally applicable. For example, in the case of

Table 1. Level of Activity in the Home: Comparison of Level Before the
Heart Attack with Current Level at T_3. Patient Report.
By Physician Recovery Rating of Patient at T_3.
In Percent. (Married Patients Only)

Rating of Activity Level: T_3 Compared with Before Heart Attack	Physician Recovery Rating			Total Reporting
	Full	Partial	Limited	
More	10.0	1.9	3.8	7.3
Same	25.4	13.2	--	19.2
Less	64.6	84.9	96.2	73.5
Total N	130	53	26	209*
Percent	100.0	100.0	100.0	100.0

* N includes (a) married patients (b) who had been rated by their
physicians at T_3 and (c) who responded to the question in one of the
three categories indicated.

[On Chi-square, p<.04; gamma = .27]

persons of great wealth, who travel a great deal, or who
are not manually oriented, it is unreasonable to expect
that their participation in chores will be substantial. The
millionaire is not likely to spend his time doing repair
work. On this point we should note that the proportion
of upper class persons in the total study population is
relatively small, and the question thus has some application to the major segment of the study group.

In broad terms, the weight of the evidence provides
some important indications of fundamental change in
one sphere of the traditional male role in the household.
It implies as well a possible increase in passivity and
assignment of former roles to others, in line with change
in health level. This trend is of interest in terms of its
implications for self perception by the patient and the
way his role is perceived by others in the household. In
many households, particularly those with the sickest
men, the role of father and husband has been substan-

tially altered, insofar as traditional male activity is concerned.

Illness and Its Influence on Members of the Family

In what ways did the illness of the husband and father influence the lives of other members of the family?

At the T_2 stage we asked each respondent, "Aside from yourself, which one of the members of your family has had to change his or her life the most because of your illness?" Although this format was directed toward the designation of individual family members, a considerable proportion of the married men—33 percent—responded, "no one." In response to a similar open-ended question at T_3, moreover, the percentage replying in the same manner was somewhat larger—44 percent. Thus, a considerable proportion of patients did not feel that other family members were significantly affected by the illness. Whether this was denial or a realistic perception can only be hypothesized.

Among the remainder of married patients, at both stages, as expected, the majority mentioned their wives as having to change the most. Of the total population, these numbered 63 percent at T_2 and 51 percent at T_3. At one year after the heart attack there was a rather predictable relationship between illness level and perceived influence upon the wife. Among married patients, who were rated by their physicians on the Recovery Index, the men given "limited" or "partial" ratings by their physicians responded in higher proportions that their wives had had to make changes than those with "full" recovery ratings—(65, 59 and 46 percent, respectively). At T_2 it was not possible to assess this variable in terms of level of illness of the patient, since all had been newly discharged from the hospital.

Finally, among those at each stage who did not

designate either their wives or "no one," most mentioned their children, and a few indicated other relatives in the home. This segment of respondents constituted a relatively small percentage of the total respondents, however.

Changes Made by Wives: A Report on Patient Perceptions at Two Stages

The types of changes which wives had to make during the year, as they were reported by the married men in the study population, can now be examined. In so doing, however, some caution in interpretation is desirable because of some minor difference in methods of questioning at the T_2 and T_3 stages.[2]

In responding to the open-ended questions about changes, most patients did not indicate multiple areas in which wives had had to alter their lives. Among the married population as a whole at T_2 (N = 306), for example, 35 percent mentioned one change only, while 27.5 percent mentioned more than one change. The majority in this latter category were noting two changes rather than a series. The maximum number—as indicated by two men in the entire study group—was four change areas. Further, a substantial proportion noted that their wives had made no changes whatever.

A pertinent question here concerns the extent to which the appearance of changes in the lives of the wives of patients is related to social or demographic variables. One may easily hypothesize that burdens of change will fall heaviest upon particular sub-segments of the population. No significant associations with any such social or demographic variables were found, however.

At one year after the heart attack, the volume of changes reported as having been made by the wife is similar in pattern to that following the hospitalization.

Among a population of 259 married respondents at T_3, 43 percent reported one change, and 30.5 percent reported two or more changes. One-fourth—27 percent—reported no changes. As in the previous interview, the majority of those wives perceived as making two or more changes actually were in the category of two changes. Few noted more than that. Four changes—the highest number—were noted by only several men.

The responses of the 259 married men at T_3 were also compared with their earlier reports concerning their wives at one month following their first hospitalization. Within this group, the report of changes at T_3 was different from T_2 for 57 percent of them. We find that 34 percent of the total reported an increase in number of changes, while 22 percent reported a decrease. The number of changes noted by 43 percent was identical at both T_2 and T_3. Thus, the percentage reporting increase is about 12 percent larger than that reporting decrease. While these data, once again, do not show any massive shift in the number of changes made by the wives, it is clear that for those who did change, the net direction was upward. The meaning of these data in terms of influence of the illness upon family life can perhaps best be noted through the examination of the specific areas in which changes were reported.

Areas of Change Among Family Members

At both the T_2 and T_3 interviews, the patients were asked for a description of the ways in which the persons noted had changed. These were all open-ended questions. The responses were then coded individually into a series of category areas, as indicated in Table 2. Table 2 presents the responses to the open-end question in order of frequency of mention.

Table 2.   Changes in Life of Wife Reported by Patient as a Result of His
Illness.   At T_2 and T_3.   Married Patients Only.   In Percent.

Selected Change Areas*	T_2	T_3	Gamma** (Stability of Response from T_2 to T_3)
Increase in wife's responsibility for family maintenance and household activities	27.4	19.3	.42
Increase in protectiveness and amount of care given patient	15.6	26.2	.58
Increase in wife's anxiety, worry, insecurity	6.5	31.3	.02
Changes in wife's social activities (i.e., reduction)	6.5	7.3	--†
Changes in job plans and employment arrangements	7.8	9.1	--†
Number of change areas reported:			
More than one	27.5	30.5	
One	35.2	42.9	.43
None	37.3	26.6	
Total N	306	259	

* Listing does not include areas for which responses were too few to
permit reporting comparisons.   Percentages are not cumulative, as some
men made more than one response.

** Gamma is based on a sub-group consisting of those married men who
responded at both T_2 and T_3 stages.   It indicates for these men the
association between their responses at the two stages.   The column
omits those men who made no reference to changes in their wives at
either stage as well as those who were part of the case loss group at
T_3.   Final item on change areas is an exception and includes those men
who responded at two stages, whether or not they indicated that their
wives had made any changes in their lives as a result of the illness.

† Not calculated because of insufficient numbers.

At T_2

As the rankings in the table show, at T_2 the change most frequently noted was that of increased responsibility for family maintenance and the management of household routines. This category covers such changes as more active role in disciplining the children and increases in heavy housework, shopping activities, and decision-making. Included also are changes in household routines managed by the wife, such as family diet, arrangement of more regular rest times, sleeping times, and similar matters. About 16 percent of married patients also indicated that the wife had become more protective, keeping the patient from troubling household situations and seeing to it that he obeyed the physician's instructions. At the lower end of the list are two items which indicate that relatively few of the men noted that the wife's anxiety had increased or that her social relationships outside the home had been altered. Though the numbers are too small to be included in the list, it should be noted that several men indicated that their spouses had had to change job plans or that they had changed their own health habits and practices, e.g., giving up smoking, changing their diet, etc.

Thus at T_2, the early period of the study year, among those wives who reportedly changed, the principal areas involved changes of role. These included the assumption of greater responsibility for management and direction in the home as well as the protection of the husband from conditions which might affect his health. Showing lowest percentages were items which pertained to psychological changes in the individual, each as anxiety level, and to social activities and job plans.

It is useful to emphasize that considerable proportions of men did not report these changes in their wives—or any changes at all. Aside from the first item, three-quarters or more of the population of married men did not indicate change on any of the areas listed.

It is likely, of course, that a direct question on each item—rather than an open-ended one—would have elicited higher positive response. But these data as they stand tell us something about what patients perceive as salient. And for most, changes in their wives as a result of the illness were not of immediate note or concern.

At T_3

At one year after the heart attack, however, we see a somewhat different picture in regard to areas of change. At that time, the proportion of men who report changes in their wives in the area of role performance has gone into a downward trend. (See Table 2, Column 2.) An interesting finding here is that the reporting of change in this area is not related to the present health rating of the patient as seen by the physician. Cross-tabulations with physician ratings revealed no significant relationships. What this may mean is that the initial fact of illness at the beginning of the year set in motion certain role reformulations in the household and that these are present one year after the hospitalization regardless of the patient's current health level.

Another finding at one year is that higher proportions of patients reported that their wives had become more anxious (31 percent). Whether this was a valid rating in the clinical sense, or whether this was merely the result of the men having greater awareness of their wives' feelings, the net effect seems clear. The men, in a considerable proportion, now had a particular contingency with which they must deal in one way or another—the anxiety of their wives and the problems in relationships which are typically associated.

Following up this finding, we explored how the appearance of anxiety in wives was reported by individuals at both T_2 and T_3. At the beginning of the year, 20 men in the total population of married men indicated this trait in their wives as a change in connection with the illness. About half of these no longer mentioned this at T_3, however. It seems useful to underline that while nearly one-third of the married men were reporting this trait in their wives at T_3, most had not previously noted it in the earlier interview.

This perceived anxiety in the wives is not significantly related to the actual health rating of the husbands at the end of the year. Moreover, additional investigation was carried out to determine the relationship of anxiety in wives to the incidence of hospitalization during the year, as well as to the appearance of additional symptoms and illness which was clinically significant but did not require hospitalization. This inquiry sought, in other words, to determine whether perception of the wife's anxiety at the end of the year was related to the husband's reported severity of health level during the year. The results were negative.

In one sense, these results conform to what is an inherent feature of anxiety—that it does not necessarily vary according to level of real danger or threat. The negative results show that regardless of health level of their husbands, wives became more anxious, or were perceived to be more anxious by their husbands.

Aside from the issue of change in family members as a result of the illness, we can also raise the related question: did those men whose wives were troubled with anxiety do less well in terms of health level than those whose wives were not? In other words, does living with an apparently anxious wife make a difference in the health of the cardiac patient? The data presented here already answer the question within the context of our measures. There is no statistical relationship between reported anxiety of the wife and the patient's health level, the physician rating or other measures of morbidity. We should like to know, however, how much the emotional change in the wife influenced the atmosphere of the home, the marital relationship and the psychological well-being of the patient. This is an aspect of the recovery process to which these empirical data point and which should be the subject of further research.

Perceived Influence on Children

Other family members involved in major ways with the illness of the patients are their children. This is not an insignificant group in terms of their number and degree of interaction with patients. For example, 91 percent of the total study group had children. Further, most had children living in the household with them. At the time of their initial admission to hospital, 70 percent of the married patients were living in households with both wife and children. The question of influence upon children, therefore, deals mainly with persons in close daily contact as household members. It deals only secondarily with a group of adult offspring who may be married and have households of their own.

As part of the series of questions concerning the influence of illness on household members, patients were asked at T_3 directly, "In what main ways do you think your illness has affected your children?" In the total population of married men with children, approximately two-thirds indicated that their children had *not* been affected by the illness.

Among that third who reported effects on the children, however, several principal themes were evident. First, men noted an increase in protectiveness and care in their children (N = 34). The children were described as being more attentive to their father, more obedient, more concerned with not disturbing him. Second, an increase in anxiety among the children was reported ($N = 31$). This was described in various terms, such as worry about the prognosis for the illness, about finances and about the future.

A third factor, mentioned by 22 men, was that their children were now more active in helping around the house and had increased their responsibility for family maintenance and household activities. Other items mentioned by several men were reduction in parent-child activities, alterations in educational plans, and changes in patterns of spending and in life style. As in the case of other variables, it is difficult to reduce overlapping in our classification of data. While in some persons an increase in protectiveness may be a response to a real situation, in others it may be primarily an expression of anxiety. Hence, the particular classifications must be evaluated in this light. Nevertheless, it must be noted that any response was recorded by only a minority of the total population of men with children. For the most part, the patients did not recognize, did not perceive, or did not choose to report any major impact of the illness on their children at one year.

This picture at one year after the heart attack repeats with some added emphasis the pattern evident at T_2. Although the question was framed in a somewhat different manner at T_3, there is little to suggest that at T_2 a large number of the patients had been concerned or impressed by the influence of the illness upon their children. At T_2, only 18 percent of the married men with children noted that their children had changed their lives in one way or another because of the illness.

The main response at T_2 was that children had increased their activity in regard to household tasks. ($N = 21$). Secondly, 11 men reported that their children had increased their protectiveness and concern. Only three men mentioned anxiety, insecurity or the unsettled emotional state of their children. Most of the others, in groups of several or less, noted such matters as potential changes in job plans, reduction in social activities because of changed financial condition of the family, etc.

Thus, at one year after the first heart attack, despite the varied histories of patients in regard to health level during the year, only a minority of the patients who were parents reported changes in their children. A main change was in the area of family roles, particularly involving assisting in the home and in taking on new responsibilities. Only a small percentage of the men at T_3 felt there were emotional changes in their children because of the illness. According to the interview data, it was primarily the wife who was affected by the illness, if anyone in the immediate family was. It was she who had to change roles or deal with her emotional state.

Changes in Role: Wife as Overseer of Activity

Perhaps the trend among patients toward doing less in the home was influenced by their wives. Many wives sought to oversee the activities of their husbands and to shield them from strain or from exertion. Some indications of this protective attitude may be seen in responses to the question, "Has your wife been making an effort to keep you from doing more than you should or to keep you from exerting yourself?"

At T_2, one month after discharge from the hospital, a relatively large proportion of the married sub-sample answered in the affirmative (90 percent). Moreover, this assessment of their wives' role persisted. At the end of the study year, 82 percent of the respondents still answered in the same way as they had at T_2.

There were only slight changes in pattern. Of those

who had answered in the affirmative at T_2, 13 percent ($N = 29$) indicated that their wives were no longer making an effort to restrict them. On the other hand, 16 men who had earlier given a negative answer reported at T_3 that their wives had been making an effort at restricting their overactivity. Only seven men in the entire group of married men stated at both T_2 and T_3 that their wives made no effort to restrict them. Thus, the evidence here suggests perception of the role of the wife as a guide and a limiter of behavior, protective and restrictive.

Further, regardless of the level of health of the individual men at the end of the year, this perception of their wives had not altered significantly. The population of married men at T_3 was compared in terms of the three categories of ratings by their physicians. When this was done, no significant differences were found between the men in regard to how they answered the question concerning restriction by their wives. Nor were there other significant relationships between the perceived restrictive role of the wife and other variables, such as age, education, occupation, or social status level.[3] The lack of finding of correlates does not mean, of course, that relationships do not exist, though they were not indicated by our measures.

Regardless of the basis for the data, however, it is apparent that wives and husbands were interacting in somewhat altered roles following the event of illness—that the husband was now someone subject to being watched over and guided by his wife for his own protection and that the wives were now assuming a new guidance role to keep their husbands from doing damage to themselves by overexertion and strain. The fact that husbands perceived and reported this aspect of their relationship in such large proportions even at one year after the first heart attack may provide some indication that some key aspects of the relationship had changed as a consequence of the illness.

ILLNESS IN THE FAMILY:
THE ISSUE OF INTERACTIVE EFFECTS

Illness of Other Family Members

In the ongoing life of a family, illness is one of the normal contingencies. In this section, we now consider the illness experience of other members of the family during the study year. There are at least three principal reasons for turning to this question. One concerns the nature of the total burdens and stresses which were placed upon the family by illness during the year. A second relates to a matter relevant to our purpose of documenting the experience and social environments of the patient following the first heart attack. While he was ill and recovering, what were the possible areas of concerns and stresses he might feel, and how might they interfere with his recovery?

A third basis links to some common hypotheses concerning the illness process. The introduction of a major stressor, one can speculate, may create loads upon other family members which may result in illness and which may even exacerbate the patient's condition. According to this viewpoint, illness in one family member may have a deteriorative effect, with the stresses introduced being expressed in illness of other members (Dohrenwend and Dohrenwend, 1969; Holmes et al., 1957; Klein et al., 1967; Myers et al., 1972; Pless et al., 1972; Rahe, 1969; Rahe et al., 1967; Pratt, 1976). An opposing hypothesis can be cited to maintain that stress introduced into the family setting serves to *integrate* the family—that there is now a focus and outlet for other family anxieties and problems. Hence this hypothesis would suggest that the level of illness in other family members would be less manifest following the patient's heart attack. Although our data can provide no ready test to deal conclusively with either of these hypotheses, the materials furnish some interesting empirical information concerning level of family illness.

At the T_2 interview we collected information concerning members of the household who had been seriously ill during the year previous to the patient's hospitalization, as well as information on the nature of the illness. Since our interest is in continuity over the year, we report here solely on data on a "select study group"—those men who participated in all three stages of the interview program (N = 259).[4] Of this group, 39 men (about 15 percent) indicated that there had been serious illness in the family before the hospitalization of the patient at T_1.

At T_3 a similar question was asked, this time concerning illness in other family members during the study year. In that interview 25 of the original 39 (about two-thirds) indicated that there had been no additional illness in the family. An additional 57 men who had *not* reported illness at T_2, however, indicated at the T_3 interview that someone had been ill subsequently. These latter men constitute 22 percent of all married men at T_3.

At the time of T_3, 71 respondents identified members of their households who had been ill with serious ailments during the previous year. Among these, about two-thirds cited their wives. About one-fourth more cited their children. The remaining minor percentages indicated their parents, inlaws, siblings, or other relatives in the household. Most of the 71 men reported on only a single additional person who had been ill besides themselves. Among those who did not (four persons), combinations of wife and children were reported. These data are similar to the distributions reported concerning illness in the household in the year previous to the heart attack.

In sum, the data indicate that additional illness in the family existed for a considerable portion of the study population. First, there were 14 men who reported illness in others at two points in time—both before their own illness and after their admission to hospital. These men, in combination with the 57, constitute a sizable grouping which had to cope with additional illness over the year. They are over one-fourth of the select study group (27.5 percent) reporting on serious illness in other family members.

On the issue of stress and the spread of illness, the data on the "select study group" provide some interesting themes.[5] In 57 families in which there had been no illness in the year before the first heart attack of the male, there was now illness. If we take as a group only those married men who reported illness-free families during the year previous to the heart attack, (N = 220), this means that one-fourth (26 percent) had families with new illness following the heart attack.

On the other hand, among those who had reported illness in household members in the year previous to the heart attack, most (N = 25) indicated that in the study year itself no one other than they was ill. Thus, it would appear that for this group there was no major recurrence of illness among family members following the heart attack of the male. In fact, two-thirds of those ill the previous year remained free of major illness during the study period.

Consider now the third question: the illness of the man as a "stress trigger." Given the data on the pre-study year, does it seem reasonable that stress in the family after the heart attack was the trigger for additional illness? First, it is useful to note that 188 families—almost three-fourths of the select study group—reported no new illness during the study year. Second, while 15 percent reported illness in the year previous to the study, the percentage of families with new illness was 27 percent. Further, a number of those with previous illness no longer reported this after the heart attack of the man. Does the difference in incidence of illness in the family between the two years—about 12 percent—constitute a significant finding? From the statistical standpoint, it does not.

Perhaps one possible lead concerning the family burdens imposed by illness in other household members can be derived from the subjective evidence of the heart patients. At T_3 each man was interviewed concerning whether the illness of others interfered with his own recovery, and in what way it did so. Of the total group for which the question was relevant, approximately 90 percent answered that such illness had not interfered. Thus, it would appear from this evidence that among this group, and for the remaining population without family illness as well, the fact of illness in the family was perceived as playing no significant negative part in the recovery or rehabilitation process of the patient.

ILLNESS SITUATION AND LIFE PROBLEMS

Influence of the Illness on Family Life: The View at One Year

While serious illness in a key family member may often exacerbate problems within the family or may create new ones, there is little to indicate that this happened within families of this study population. According to reports by the patients themselves, where the illness presented significant problems, it was mostly in areas other than family relationships or in the situations of family members. How the problems relate to those of the family specifically can be seen in findings from both the T_2 and the T_3 interviews.

At T_3 patients were asked a general question concerning problems which had existed prior to the illness and which had been exacerbated by the illness experience. The question was, "Everyone has problems, and sometimes when people become sick some of those problems are made more difficult to deal with. In your own case, has your illness made the problems you had before more difficult to deal with?" About a fifth of the patients answered in the affirmative.

It should be clear that at T_3 we are asking for recall going beyond a year, to the period before the heart attack, and that we are asking for an assessment of continuity of problems over an extended period. While limited in depending on extended recall, such an approach does provide some subjective assessments of the effects of the illness on the quality of life, *as perceived by the patient.*

Among the 20 percent who did report an exacerbation of problems by the illness, few noted that any of these dealt with family matters or family issues. In fact, in regard to their relationships with wives, only a few patients had anything to report. One indicated that his wife's emotional difficulties had been made worse by the illness. Several others indicated that their marital adjustment had become worse, and that they had more conflict and disagreements. With regard to their children, three men noted that the illness had increased their difficulties in providing financial support, particularly in regard to furnishing funds for their education. Three men mentioned that their previous disciplinary problems with children had been made more difficult by the illness. Thus, only these small numbers of patients had anything to say about the impact of illness on family problems *per se*. Their major concerns were with problems of work, such as job advancement, meeting job pressures, and the like, and with their declining capacity to perform at a satisfactory physical level.

In another open-ended question at one year, we asked patients what they saw as their major problems for the future. Here a slightly higher proportion of patients saw problems—27 percent. Once again, however, only a few mentioned issues pertaining to family matters. Three men cited problems related to their wives. The several who had noted difficulties during the year as a result of the illness had presumably mastered them and did not see them as continuing into the future. The picture was not substantially different with respect to children. At the end of the year, 13 men noted that they were concerned about their ability to provide financially for the education of their children. It appears that the issue of finances loomed as a main concern to these men, and there were few interpersonal problems with family members attributed to the illness.

As in the case of the previous question concerning pre-illness problems, the men were directly concerned with future problems which involve the family only in a general sense: the issues of survival and maintaining their health, of finding appropriate work, their future capacity to be employed, and obtaining sufficient funds to support their family. Relationships and roles, and future education of children were of lesser concern.

Assessment at T_2: Perception of Problems to Come

The preceding data at one year are similar in pattern to those evident at T_2. At T_2, men were asked the same question as above: whether the problems before the illness had been made more difficult by it. At that time 21 percent responded in the affirmative. At the T₂ period the first hospitalization and the first shock of illness were relatively fresh. Therefore, it would seem that at this time of high emotion and uncertainty there would be reflections on the nature of family relationships. If there were, however, these did not appear as substantial problems in the interviews.

What were these matters as they pertained to the family? Only eight of the married men noted that their relationships with their wives had been made more difficult by the illness—a number which was subsequently reduced over the year. With regard to children, continuing problems of discipline were noted by only three men. As at the later period, the chief problems reported to have been made more difficult by the illness were those relating to finances (insufficient income, bills) and those relating to work (finding employment, meeting the requirements of the job).

These open-ended questions give perspective on the illness, and it is likely that higher percentages of men would have reported on family problems if they had been asked with direct, fixed alternative questions. In choosing this approach, we have avoided forcing people to express opinions even when they have none (Converse, 1963).

The Family: Financial Concerns and the Employment of Wives

A recurring theme throughout the previous sections is the concern of patients with matters of basic family economics: problems of income, holding a job, supporting the family, and having sufficient funds to educate the children. It is in this area, perhaps, that the most fundamental threats to family integration and quality of life occurred during the first year after the occurrence of the heart attack. Since these matters have already been covered in Chapter 4, we need only note them briefly here in this discussion of the family.

As the earlier findings show, the economic burdens of the illness seem to fall most upon two groups distinguished within the study population: (a) those who had recurrences of illness during the year and (b) those in the lower socioeconomic groups. Within these groups were the greatest problems of adequate income, insecurities about employment and future capacity for work, as well as changes in patterns of spending and those aspects of life style influenced by economic capacity. Further, as we have just seen, these financially related problems were reflected also in the expressed anxieties and concerns of the patients. Among those who reported problems in their lives, the most salient concerned work, income and finance, rather than on more subtle aspects of changes in role relationships, shifts in the authority structure in the home and alteration of the emotional tone.

Further, as noted in the earlier chapter, the illness did not lead to any significant change in the proportion of working wives. Before the illness of the man, wives in a substantial percentage of the families were employed (43 percent of married couples). This was a pattern which was not related to social status or socioeconomic level. Regardless of health history of the men during the year, the pattern of wife employment did not change. Many variables influence whether or not wives are in the labor market: economic need, interest factors, and stage of the family life cycle. In families where the wife was not previously working and where there was economic need, it appears that adjustments were made through altering spending patterns and life style rather than through the wife's entrance into the labor market.

THE MARRIAGE RELATIONSHIP:
TWO PERSPECTIVES

We now turn to the question of change in some relationships in the home and to the possible influence of the illness upon them. Here we center on two issues: (1) what happens to the marriage relationship over time following the first crisis of serious illness and (2) in what ways is the marriage affected by the occurrence of subsequent ill health in the husband over the course of the year? These are broad and complex matters. To deal with some limited areas for purposes of this report, however, two indices of selected aspects of the marriage are employed. These are: (1) level of reported consensus or disagreement on issues and (2) appraisal by the patient of his own "happiness" in the marriage, as well as the "happiness" of his wife.

Marital Consensus and Illness Level

In line with our interest in the impact of illness upon family life, we developed information from the interviews concerning the husband-wife relationship. The question of influence of stress upon the husband-wife relationship is one for which research thus far has produced conflicting answers. From the limited research literature and from the mass of speculation and theorizing, contrary cases may be made which indicate that stress in itself may be integrative or it may be deteriorative in marital situations (Aguilera and Messick, 1974; Croog, 1970; Rapoport, 1963). Given this mixed picture as well as our purposes of documenting the illness experience of the study population, we collected information dealing with one aspect of the marital relationship: the pattern of consensus or disagreements between husband and wife. In this section we report on patterns of marital disagreement and on areas of change during the year following the first heart attack.

At both the T_2 and T_3 interviews husband and wife were questioned concerning the occurrence of disagreement on a series of common issues and areas. The listing was derived from previous scales developed by Burgess and Wallin in connection with their work on prediction of marital satisfaction (Burgess and Wallin, 1953). The full set of items employed is reported in Table 3.

At T_2 and T_3 the respondents were asked, "Every marriage has its agreements and disagreements. We would like to know how often you and your wife disagree in regard to each of the following things." Each item on the listing was reviewed separately. The respondent was presented the following alternative possibilities: "often disagree," "disagree once in a while," "never disagree." ("Not applicable" and "not relevant" categories were also noted.) The materials were then coded in terms of presence or absence of disagreement. That is, those who indicated that they disagreed on an item "often" or "once in a while" were classified as having given a positive response. Positive disagreement was coded as such when both husband and wife indicated disagreement, or when one spouse only gave an indication.

The second criterion was used on the assumption that reporting of disagreement by one spouse was sufficient evidence of lack of consensus on the matter. The spouses, in effect, were not in agreement as to whether they disagreed. This method was used partly to compensate for unconscious denial and repression. In some areas, for example, such as expression of affection or religious matters, it was assumed that some of the disagreement might not be expressed or verbalized. One spouse might consciously note the presence of conflict while the other was unaware of it, or repress the knowledge to avoid confrontation.

Data were examined through analysis of individual items as well as through use of a Marital Disagreement Index. This index was devised through the classification of responses into a three category scale as follows: low disagreement: citation of zero through four items; medium: citation of five through seven items; and high: citation of eight or more. Initial classification of the data into three categories at T_2 led to the following distributions: low: 38 percent; medium: 38 percent; and high: 23 percent. This distribution was carried out so that the number of items in each category might be relatively similar, i.e., four items for the first, three for the second, and three for the third. On a 12-item listing, no one reported zero, and at the other extreme no one indicated 12 items.

In focusing on consensus within the marriage over time, these materials deal with reported conflict and have little to do with level of marital satisfaction. Other variables deal with this, as will be seen. Some measure of disagreement is inevitable in marriage, and of course some disagreement may be functional and constructive in the relationship. It is an indication that spouses are able to express strong feelings to one another—that they can express individuality.[6]

One feature of the data on disagreement is the relative stability over the course of the study year. In Table 3, percentages are shown indicating the proportion of married couples for whom the report concerning disagreement in an area was the same at both T_2 and T_3. The percentages, it must be emphasized, should not be interpreted as indicating disagreement, but only whether or not the same answer was given at both T_2 and T_3. The gamma scores indicate the same data in correlational form. Matters pertaining to religion, family finances, their children, and the question of where to

Table 3.   Changes in Reported Marital Disagreement on Selected Issues:
From T2 to T3.   Percent of Married Couples Reporting on Presence or
Absence of Disagreement on the Issue.

Item	(1) Reported at Both T_2 and T_3	(2) Reported at T_2; Not Reported at T_3	(3) Not Reported at T_2; Reported at T_3	Gamma Scores: Responses at T_2 and T_3*	Total N for Each Item (Husband-Wife Pairs)**
On bringing up children	50.3	18.2	9.4***	.73	159
Handling family finances	46.0	18.4	8.7	.77	196
How to spend leisure time	40.7	19.6	14.4	.57	194
Dealing with in-laws	29.7	20.9	13.2	.60	182
Demonstration of affection	20.7	18.7	11.4	.66	193
Sharing of household tasks	20.7	19.2	11.4	.64	193
Making major purchases	20.6	18.0	15.5	.54	194
Friends	20.4	25.5	12.2	.46	196
Amount of time to be spent together	14.0	16.0	16.0	.70	194
Table manners	13.3	12.8	8.2	.78	195
Where to live	7.7	8.8	10.3	.72	194
Religious matters	7.3	6.7	6.2	.86	193

* Gamma scores indicate association between responses at T_2 and T_3.
Score is based on both positive and negative responses. In other
words, it simply indicates continuity or stability of original responses of husband and wife from T_2 to T_3.

** Size of N is reduced on items for "Children" and "In-laws," where
patient reported no children or no living in-laws. Other minor
variations are due to non-response or "undecided."

*** Percentages in the first three columns do not add to 100, as data are
omitted on negative responses reported at both T_2 and T_3.

live ranked among the areas on which responses were most stable.

The main portion of the population did not alter its response on each item over the course of the year, and only a minority segment of couples indicated changes. Columns 2 and 3 show those percentages of the total for whom the data at the two stages show change. Column 2 gives the percentages who indicated disagreement on an item at T_2 but not at T_3. Column 3 shows the obverse, i.e., couples who originally had no report of disagreement at T_2 but who did indicate disagreement at the end of the year.

On the whole, the data in the two columns show remarkable similarity in level of percentage. One interesting point, however, is that for nine of the 12 items, the percentage of persons who no longer mentioned an item at the end of the year is greater than the percentage who noted a new item of disagreement at the end of the year. In no instance is the difference in percentage statistically significant. These data, insofar as they show pattern, indicate that there was no marked trend toward greater or lesser disagreement on any individual item during the year following initial illness.

While reported level of disagreement on *individual* items remained relatively stable, a somewhat different pattern may be seen when the *total number* of items are considered. Although consideration of individual items tells about specific areas, it does not inform about the total volume of disagreements. In many ways the total volume may be a more important statistic, for it moves away from consideration of specific issues to indicate level of reported tension, as seen through net disagreements.

Turning to the Index of Marital Disagreement, several points can be noted. First, when categorized into the three classes of low, medium and high, about half the population remained in the same group from T_2 to T_3. Of the remainder, 40 percent of the population moved from a higher to a lower category, indicating fewer items reported. The minority proportion increased (12 percent). Thus, these data, though perhaps crude indicators of subtle phenomena, seem to show that the main pattern was stability in disagreement level coupled with a tendency toward decrease in number of items. The study year, according to these reports, was apparently not one of exacerbated marital conflict.

What of the issue of possible association of the health level of the patient with level of marital disagreement? At the end of the study year the data show little relationship between health level and the reported degree of marital disagreement at that time. Using the physician's assessment of the patients, we compared married patients classified according to three categories of current functional status: full, partial, and limited.[7] There was a slight tendency for men with other than full recovery, i.e., classified as "partial" or "limited" to score high on the Marital Disagreement Index. The difference amounts to only 10 percent above the full recovery group, however, and was not statistically significant. Similarly, when the rehospitalized married men were compared with the nonrehospitalized, there were no significant statistical differences in marital disagreement level.

According to these data it does not seem that level of marital disagreement is meaningfully related in either a positive or negative sense to recovery status. In more literal terms, marriages in which the husbands are the most healthy do not report disagreeing less than those where the husband continues to have serious illness problems. Nor do the data on the rehospitalized versus the nonrehospitalized support an "integration hypothesis" viewpoint, i.e., that illness stress brings the family together, reducing the likelihood of marital conflicts.

Reported Happiness in Marriage and Level of Illness

In the preceding section, we focused upon the Marital Disagreement Index as a means of assessing the possible positive and negative impact of the illness upon the marital relationship. Another way of exploring the effects of the illness upon the patients' marriages is to analyze patient reports of their marital happiness and that of their spouses. We are interested particularly in the stability of the reports during the first year after the myocardial infarction and the possible relationship of reported marital happiness to patient health level.

Among the many possible measures of the complex relationships in marriage, one obvious and elementary measure is the subjective feeling of the participants. While science may dictate that we should apply various measures to tap specified dimensions, one may also obviously gain some critical information by simply asking a husband or wife "How happy is the marriage?" Further, one can note how these subjective reports change over time.

At both T_2 and T_3 we asked the patient, "Everything considered, how happy would you say your marriage has been?" A set of fixed alternative responses were set forth: "very happy, happy, average, unhappy, very unhappy." In addition, the same question was asked of the patient in regard to his wife, so that some notion of the cognitive world of the patient might be discerned. Here the phrasing was slightly different: "Everything considered, would you say your wife has found your marriage to be very happy, happy, average, unhappy, or very unhappy?"

At one year after the first heart attack, there appears to be no relationship between the patient's appraisal of his marriage and the health rating which he was given in the physician reports. For example, while 54 percent of the men rated as having made "full" recovery characterized their marriage as "very happy," so too did 50 percent of those classed as having made "partial" or "limited" recovery. A similar pattern is evident when patients' responses concerning their wives' happiness in the marriage is appraised. No relationship appears between health level of the patient and the reported perception of his wife's feelings.

Despite the differing health experiences of the previous year, the ratings of the marriages remained relatively stable, as seen when the T_2 responses are compared with T_3. Comparing the husband's appraisals at T_2 and at T_3, there appears a correlation (gamma) of .72. Comparing his appraisals of his wife's happiness in the marriage at T_2 and T_3, the correlation if .67. Among those patients who changed their appraisal, the percentage moving up is similar to the percentage moving down. In regard to the patients' ratings of their own marital happiness, 16 percent noted an increase in happiness at T_3, and 14 percent reported a decrease. In regard to the patients' ratings of their wives' marital happiness, comparable figures were 19.5 percent and 24 percent.

It must be remembered that the subjects in our study are, for the most part, settled couples with a long period of life together and of sharing experiences. Half had been married for at least 21 years. In the entire group, three-quarters had been married for 16 years or more. Ninety percent of the marriages had produced children. Hence, viewing the evidence of long-term relationships and adjustments worked out over time, it is understandable that the illness did not produce changes in appraisals of marital happiness nor in the quality of the marital relationship.

Who is to Blame? Wives? Children? Perceptions of Etiology

Some further indications of stresses in family life may be seen in perceptions by husbands and wives of the causes of the initial heart attack. As we have noted elsewhere (See Chapter 1, Note 3), patients and wives were asked at both T_2 and T_3 to rate a series of items in regard to their importance as contributing to the etiology of the heart attack. Among these items were "problems with wife," and "upsetting problems with children."

Among the married men, nearly 20 percent at T_2 cited problems with the wife as "important." Among those with children, about 25 percent cited problems with children as important in the etiology. Among the wives, there were similar perceptions. Thus, 21 percent cited problems with the wife as being important and 27 percent mentioned that problems with children were important.

It is interesting to note that the husbands and wives who responded in this way were not all members of the same marital pairs. It appears that in 30 percent of all the married couples, either the husband, the wife, or both partners cited problems in their marital relationships as being important in causing the heart attack. Similarly, in 37 percent of families with children, either the husband, the wife, or both partners cited problems with children as an important factor in the etiology of the heart attack. Further, these figures were virtually duplicated at T_3, one year after the heart attack, indicating persistence of these beliefs and feelings.

Given other evidence available in the interviews, it is likely that a number of other men and women felt the same way on these matters but chose not to report these feelings at that particular point in the interview schedule. These data imply a great deal about the nature of the marital relationship as it relates to the illness. The suspicions of the husbands, their feelings of hostility toward their wives, the possible feelings of guilt on the part of the wives—these may be part of the underlying emotional themes in the family which our data reflect. Similar comments might be made about the emotional tone of the parent-child relationship as this relates to the illness of the father.

USE OF RESOURCES AND SUPPORTS: FAMILY AND NON-FAMILY

In this section we return to another main theme of this report: the "armory of resources" of patients and the ways in which these resources are used. Here we move outside the nuclear family of the patients and turn attention to members of his larger family, the extended kin group. The purpose here is to describe the type and nature of support and assistance provided by kin. In addition, we consider the varied supports provided by friends and neighbors. We examine the role of these non-family members as surrogate or quasi-kin during illness.

Consideration of kin and non-kin sources of support links into another, larger question concerning types of resources available and used in a modern, industrialized society. According to one prominent view, under conditions of urbanization and industrialization kinship units become highly specialized, and other institutional structures take over those functions which are commonly performed by families in non-industrialized societies (Linton, 1949; Ogburn, 1934; Parsons, 1943; Parsons and

Bales, 1955). On the American scene this phenomenon has been associated with the relative structural isolation of the family. According to this thesis, members of nuclear families tend to rely more upon the formal institutions and agencies of the society for support rather than upon the kinship unit.

On the other hand, evidence from various recent studies shows that even in the context of an industrialized society the extended family is a viable resource, often as a result of rapid communication and transportation (Adams, 1968; Litwak, 1960; Sussman, 1965; Sussman and Burchinal, 1962). In fact, some increasing evidence indicates that in times of disaster, individuals turn first to family members and close friends. Relief agencies and public institutions rank last in the hierarchy of preference and use (Quarantelli, 1960).

The role of friends and neighbors as sources of support during times of stress constitutes another unresolved issue which must be considered in evaluations of the family as a resource (Litwak and Szelenyi, 1969; Useem et al., 1960; Zimmerman and Cervantes, 1960, Chen and Cobb, 1960; Moriyama et al., 1971). Some formulations point to the primacy of the family as a first line of support, with friends and neighbors serving as supplements rather than as substitutions (Rosow, 1967). How these varied resource groups operate in the case of illness crises has rarely been systematically studied, and there are few data concerning the factors which are related to the providing of different patterns of aid or support by family and non-family resources. Some notable reports have been filling these gaps in recent years, although there are problems of comparability of findings (Adams, 1968; Axelrod, 1956).

One aspect of the question of use of resources in an industrial society has been discussed in Chapter 5: the degree to which patients utilize agencies and institutions.

The low level of reported usage may be idiosyncratic, of course, stemming from the unique situation of a study population with little need for institutions and agencies, and with little need for referral. Regardless of the basis for minimal use, however, it is apparent that in the case of these patients, at least, the support resources of the society were not a major factor in their illness histories. We now turn to consider the use of kin and non-kin persons as resources.

In the next paragraphs, we report data on the following: (1) Perceptions of the level of help or support furnished by various members of the kin group and by extrafamilial sources, such as neighbors and friends; (2) Variables associated with degrees of support perceived as having been given by family and non-family sources. (These variables include age of patients, educational level, social class, social interaction level, ethnic origins, and level of need as indicated by recurrence of illness crisis.) The purpose here is to examine the nature of the conditions under which family and non-family sources provide resources and support. (3) Types of help provided by members of the kin group as compared with outside sources, such as neighbors and friends.

By reporting on the three categories we draw together materials on a range of resources (family, non-family, institutional); the level of support furnished; some substantive areas of support, and the correlates of differential contribution by support sources.[8]

Some Definitions and Criteria

The data concerning help from kin and non-kin are drawn from the retrospective statements of the patients at the time of the T_3 interview. The respondents were asked to provide an assessment of the level of assistance which had been provided them by various kin and non-kin sources in connection with their illness and recovery. In addition, they were asked to indicate the types of help provided, and these were classified according to such general categories as "services provided," "moral support," and "financial aid furnished."

The category "moral support" is one which patients reported, and which we incorporated because patients apparently perceived it as a real and distinctive entity. At the same time, however, we wish to emphasize that while patients mentioned this specifically, the other two categories, "services" and "financial help," could also be classified as "moral support." In a sense, anyone who did anything for the patient which made him feel better, encouraged him, or improved his spirits, might be said to have constributed "moral support."

Persons who reported that both parents were dead or that they had no siblings are excluded from those sections of the analysis dealing with parents or siblings. In the study population of 293 respondents at T_3, the following proportions indicated having relevant kin or non-kin and made ratings of level and type of aid: parents, 44.5 percent; siblings, 87 percent; in-laws, 82 percent; other relatives, 69 percent; friends, 98 percent; and neighbors, 97 percent.

In a preliminary screening question, patients were asked to indicate how many close relatives lived within easy driving distance. Ninety-four percent indicated the presence of relatives within easy access. Though proximity may improve level of support, this is not as critical a variable as it may appear, even in the case of the small proportion who had no relatives close by. Access to travel facilities, as well as the use of the telephone and mail, tend to minimize the importance of geographical distance, and such types of aid as moral support and financial help are not necessarily contingent on face-to-face contact.

Kin and Non-kin Sources of Help

HELP SOURCES: KIN, FRIENDS, AND NEIGHBORS.   Table 4 presents patients' ratings of the degree of help which they received from kinship and non-kinship sources. As may be seen, those ranking highest in the "very helpful" category were members of the patient's own family: his siblings and his parents. In addition, the large mixed category classified as "in-laws" ranks at the same level as the family members, siblings and parents. The table also indicates that non-family resources such as "friends" rank nearly as high. Lowest of all in the rankings is the larger kin group designated as "other relatives."

Table 4.   Level of Help Reported from Kin and Nonkin Sources.   Percent.

Source	Very Helpful	Somewhat Helpful; Not too Helpful	Not Helpful At All	N
Kin				
Parents	43.6 (58)	27.8 (37)	28.6 (38)	133*
Siblings	45.7 (117)	32.8 (84)	21.5 (55)	256*
In-Laws	43.3 (103)	31.5 (75)	25.2 (60)	238*
Other Relatives	19.6 (39)	31.2 (62)	49.3 (98)	199*
Nonkin				
Friends	38.3 (110)	45.3 (130)	16.4 (47)	287
Neighbors	29.4 (83)	35.8 (101)	34.7 (98)	282

* Table excludes "Not Relevant" and "Don't Know" responses.

While these ratings appear to reaffirm the relative importance of immediate kin in performing functions of help and support, the contributions of non-kin, such as friends and neighbors, are clearly evident. In fact, it appears that friends and neighbors are even more important than the more distant kin group, "other relatives," in terms of perceived helpfulness.

Another aspect of the table which deserves note is the third column, in which are recorded responses indicating the most negative of appraisals, "not helpful at all." Here nearly 30 percent of the patients included their parents and about one-fifth included their siblings. The group which was least frequently mentioned as not helpful was friends, a fact which implies that such non-family resources, though they may not be predominant among the "very helpful," are at least a common resource.

Patterns of Assistance and Associated Variables

How do family and non-family sources of aid or support compare with each other in terms of the patterns of assistance which each provides? Patients who had responded that a particular class of individuals was "very helpful" or "somewhat helpful" were asked to specify the kinds of help which these had given. These were classified in terms of the categories reported in Table 5.

Table 5. Type of Help Reported from Kin and Nonkin Aid Sources. By Patients Reporting Significant Help from Each Category. Percent.*

Source	Services	Moral Support	Financial Aid	Base N**
Kin				
Parents	30.5	67.1	25.6	82
Siblings	34.0	71.8	21.3	177
In-Laws	34.1	73.8	13.4	164
Other Relatives	20.3	77.0	8.1	74
Nonkin				
Friends	33.6	72.5	9.5	211
Neighbors	54.8	58.0	3.2	157

* Percentages are non-cumulative, insofar as individuals may have mentioned more than one type of help from each category of kin or nonkin.

** Base N includes those cases in which a respondent indicated that persons in the category were either "Very helpful" or "Somewhat helpful."

As the data in Table 5 indicate, the type of assistance offered by persons rated as helpful varies according to kin and non-kin relationships. Within each category of persons, the item most frequently cited was "moral support." This type of aid is prominent among neighbors and friends as well as among members of both close and distant kin groups.

The second most frequently mentioned type of aid received from kin and non-kin sources rated as helpful was "services." Of those who ranked neighbors as having provided aid, a relatively high proportion (55 percent) mentioned their having provided services. Though members of the immediate family rank below neighbors on this variable, the picture is somewhat different in regard to financial aid. Among those patients who had rated parents and siblings as helpful, 26 percent mentioned parents and 21 percent mentioned siblings as having given financial aid. Few who regarded neighbors as helpful reported that they gave financial aid.

An exploration was carried out to determine whether there was significant association between several characteristics of patients and their reported receipt of particular types of aid from the several sources. Of the variables considered, only age of the patient appeared to be significantly associated with types of aid from various sources. As may be seen in Table 6, the report of financial assistance is the item most prominently associated with age. Here the data indicate an inverse association between age of patient and receipt of such aid from parents, siblings, and in-laws. In regard to moral support and receipt of services from parents, significant negative associations with age were also found. In all other instances, however, gamma scores were low, as the table indicates.

Although in general education and social class were not found to be related to types of aid from various

Table 6.   Association Between Age of Patient and Type of
Support Reported from Kin and NonKin Sources.   Gamma Scores†

Source	Services	Financial Help Offered††	Moral Support
Kin			
Parents	-.51***	-.54***	-.42***
Siblings	-.14	-.48***	.04
In-Laws	-.13	-.64***	.05
Other Relatives	-	-	.21
NonKin			
Friends	-.26*	-.42*	.11
Neighbors	-.17	-	.07

† Gamma scores are not reported for categories in which numbers
in cells were insufficient for Chi-square test.

†† The category "Financial Help Offered" includes reference to
cases in which financial aid was received as well as reported
as offered.

On Chi-square test: *p<.10
                        **p<.05
                       ***p<.01

sources, a significant negative association was found between educational level and the number of patients reporting financial aid from siblings.

Levels of Support from Aid Sources: Associated Variables

While the data in Table 4 show the perceived helpfulness of persons in the various kin and non-kin categories, these materials raise questions concerning the characteristics of those recipients who reported receiving differing degrees of help. In order to deal at least in part with these questions, we examined a series of social identity and health-status characteristics of the patients in regard to the level of help which they reported they received from each kin and nonkin source.

In Table 7 we report a series of gamma scores indicating associations between reported level of help from each source and such characteristics as age, education,

Table 7.   Association Between Characteristics of Respondents and Degree of Help from Kin and NonKin Sources. Gamma Scores.

	Parents	Siblings	In-Laws	Other Relatives	Friends	Neighbors
Reported Setbacks	.05	.06	.16	-.06	.25*	.19
Frequency of Visits[1]	.26**	.28**	.13	.19*	.28**	.38**
Age	-.60**	-.21	-.22	.05	-.12	-.12
Education	.02	-.12	-.16	-.12	-.04	.04
Social Class	.16	-.02	-.07	.02	.07	.08

Level of significance as indicated by Chi-square test: * = $p < .05$
                                                        ** = $p < .01$

[1]This item refers to frequency of visits by the patient to persons in each category.

social class, frequency of visits before illness, and whether the patient had additional needs, as indicated by illness setbacks. Table 8 presents data on the association between degree of reported help received from a single category in relation to other categories. These appear in the table as a matrix of gamma scores. The issue of ethnic origin as a possible correlate of level of help received is then discussed separately.

Illness Setbacks and the Question of Differences in Need for Help

During the course of the year a group of patients (30 percent) reported having had setbacks in their illness. These involved recurrence of symptoms, a new heart attack or occurrence of other disease. Can the pattern of aid be explained merely in terms of level of need, as indicated by the patient's report of setbacks? One simple hypothesis is that patients who do not need help do not receive it, while those who have need are more likely to receive it. Through reference to empirical data, we sought to explore whether persons in the most marked distress situation, those reporting setbacks, were more likely to report higher degrees of assistance than those who did not have setbacks.

As Table 7 shows, the reporting of setbacks generally had little association with level of help received from most sources, with the exception of the "friends" category. One might speculate from these data that regardless of the level of difficulty of the patient, family members were likely to assist him. Friends and neighbors may constitute a different case, however. Lacking the impetus of family obligations and mutual aid, they might simply respond when the situation seemed most urgent, rallying around those whose need is evident.

Pre-Illness Visiting Pattern

Among the characteristics of respondents for which gamma scores are reported in Table 7, the one most highly related to level of perceived support is visiting pattern. It appears that the greater the frequency of visits by the patient to persons in each category before his illness, the more likely he was to report a high degree of help during the recovery and rehabilitation periods. If frequency of visits may be taken as an indication of favorable interpersonal relationships, it is not unreasonable to expect that persons with whom the patient had good relations before he became ill would be most likely to help him.

One point of interest here is that there is an association between the patient's previous pattern of visiting friends and neighbors and the level of aid received from these non-kin persons. Here the gamma scores are higher than those for such kin groups as in-laws and other relatives.

Age

An item to note in Table 7 is the relationship between age of patient and level of help received. Here the highest gamma scores are found among members of the family, including parents, siblings, and in-laws, although only the score of .60 for parents is distinctive. This association may mean that the younger patients had younger parents, and these were more able to provide support than the elderly parents of older patients. Negative relationships between age of married couples and the degree of help received from parental sources have also been reported in other studies of kin network and mutual aid (Adams, 1964; Sussman and Burchinal, 1962).

Social Status

Perhaps the most unusual finding in Table 7 is the lack
of significant association between level of help reported
and either educational level or social class of the patient.
Many studies have reported differing levels of interaction and degrees of cohesion among families from varying class origins, and markedly different types of
involvement with neighbors and friends have often been
portrayed (Aldous, 1967; Shanas, 1967). There is no
apparent evidence from this patient group, however,
that social class or status is related to the level of help
received from various family and non-family sources.

Ethnic Origins

Many descriptive reports, as well as many stereotyped
statements, have appeared in the literature concerning
differential levels of cohesion of various subcultural or
ethnic groups (Cavan, 1964; Glazer and Moynihan,
1963; Winch and Greer, 1968). In an effort to screen
relevant variables which might account for levels of help
reported by patients, we also examined ethnic origins as
a factor. We decided to test specifically whether membership in a family with particular ethnic characteristics
might be related to level of help received. For this purpose the four largest ethnic groupings in the study
population were selected following procedures reported
in Chapter 1. Distributions are as follows: Irish (N = 61);
Italian (N = 47); Jewish (N = 43); and British-Old American (N = 29).

No significant differences were found between
members of these ethnic groups when compared with
each other or with the remainder of the study population in regard to level of help received from family or
non-family sources. While it is possible that there are

Table 8.   Association Between Degrees of Reported Helpfulness from Kin and NonKin Sources.   Gamma Scores.

	Parents	Siblings	In-Laws	Other Relatives	Friends	Neighbors
Parents	–	.86**	.49**	.77**	.69**	.67**
Siblings		–	.57**	.67**	.72**	.56**
In-Laws			–	.66**	.68**	.61**
Other Relatives				–	.54**	.55**
Friends					–	.78**
Neighbors						–

** p<.01 on Chi-square test.

significant variations between ethnic groups in terms of kin relations and mutual aid, these may tend to be minimized in a situation of crisis, such as serious illness.

Associations Between Degree of Help From Kin and Non-kin Sources

As may be seen in Table 8, the level of help reported as coming from any single kin or non-kin category is significantly associated with the help level from each other category. For example, those who received a high degree of aid from parents also reported a high level of aid from other kin as well as from non-kin sources. Gamma scores range from .57 to .86.

Social Integration and Levels of Support: Consideration of an Hypothesis

Among those variables reviewed here, the best predictor of level of perceived helpfulness in one category of kin or non-kin is the level of perceived helpfulness in other categories (Table 8). In other words, the degree of aid from one source was highly associated with the degree of aid from others. A second set of significant associations related pre-morbid visiting patterns to helpfulness (Table 7). These two findings combined raise the possibility that the underlying phenomenon may be the level of social integration of an individual. Individuals who are socially well integrated will, by definition, have favorable relationships with others. These are marked by solidarity, including mutual visiting and emotional and material support. Hence in severe illness these individuals may be most likely to receive aid from multiple sources, including the various kinship categories as well as friends and neighbors. In practical terms, these findings may also mean that the better integrated the individual, the higher the degree of assistance he receives, and that non-family sources are apparently as available and helpful to him as most categories of the kin group. Similar findings regarding association between integration within a kin network and aid furnished during illness have been reported by Sussman on the basis of an exploratory study (Sussman, 1965).

Perhaps more dramatic is the negative side of the relationship in Table 8, indicating as it does that those who report low helpfulness from one kin group are also likely to report minimal aid from other kin categories as well as from friends and neighbors.

Of equal interest from the sociological standpoint was the lack of association between help pattern and such variables as perceived illness setbacks, social class, and ethnic origin. In addition, an obvious hypothesis is that the degree of *need* of the patient determines how much assistance he will receive and from which sources. In our data on correlates of help patterns, patients who indicated that they had difficulties in the form of setbacks in their illness did not report a different level of help received when compared with those who did not give such indications. The issues concerning "patient needs" and their valid measurement are complex, and they clearly deserve further exploration. For the present, however, we must point out that, as far as these data are concerned, other variables appeared more closely associated to help patterns than were the "setbacks" perceived and reported by the patient.

SUMMARY

Over the course of the study year, the general picture on the whole, is one of apparent coping with the illness. Relatively minimal impact on family life is reported, except for some aspects of role performance, e.g., despite financial concerns, the percentage of working wives did not change significantly during the year. About 80 percent of patients reported that problems which had existed before their illness were not aggravated by it, and of the problems reported to be exacerbated by the illness, the majority were not family-related. No significant differences in this general pattern appeared when major age or demographic sub-groups were examined.

Some indications of notable change in role performance among family members were evident. For example, at T_2 two-thirds of the married men reported that their wives had made role changes. Most of these changes were perceived as involving greater responsibility and leadership in the home, as well as increased protectiveness of the husband. Further, about 75 percent of the patients reported a change in their own role, in the direction of a decline in the level of their activity in household tasks and duties.

Focus on the level of marital integration—as indicated by presence or absence of consensus on issues, produced several related findings. First, the level of agreement or disagreement remained stable among almost half of the families. Among those who did change in consensus levels, however, the majority reported a *decline* in disagreement over the course of the study year. Thus, it seems clear that the illness apparently did not exacerbate or increase the level of conflict between spouses. Further, those families in which the man was most seriously ill during the year did not differ from the remainder in level of consensus on issues. In other words, the subsequent level of severity of illness was not related to the marital consensus.

The effects of serious illness as a stressor or trigger for illness in other family members was examined. In this population at least, no significant data emerged pointing to an increase in illness among family members in the year after the heart attack. Nor was this particularly evident among the families of the men who were most seriously ill during the year, the rehospitalized. Other data in the chapter indicate that perhaps the main consequence for family health was the perceived increased anxiety level in wives.

Finally, the pattern of aid, as furnished by family and non-kin sources, was examined. Here it appeared that the more highly socially integrated patients received aid from more sources. Also non-kin, such as neighbors and friends, emerged as important resources in the period following hospitalization. Although it is commonly hypothesized that modern industrial institutions and organizations of the larger society are taking over many of the roles of the traditional kin groups, in this heart patient study population kin and quasi-kin played important supportive roles.

NOTES

1. See Chapter 2 for a description of the physician assessment scale.
2. At T_2, we asked those men who had mentioned their wives as having changed the most to specify and describe the changes. At T_3 we did the same. At T_2 and T_3 there were follow-up questions to the one on who had changed the most. At T_2 we asked the respondent in what ways others in the household had changed their lives because of the illness. Thus, after specifying the one who had changed the most and in what ways, he was invited to fill in on others as well. This would include his wife, if she had not already been mentioned.

   At T_3, since we wished to obtain information about the wife specifically, we asked about changes the wife had to make, following the question dealing with who had to change the most. At both stages, in coding responses, we combined answers to the questions concerning wives, so that a general picture of changes by wives would be developed, whether or not they had been specified as having changed the most. In evaluating the data concerning changes over time, one must decide whether the patterns of difference and/or similarity are due to the questions or to other factors. This point, of course, is not pertinent when the data at T_1 and T_4 are considered separately.
3. For variable measurement techniques, see Reference 4, Chapter 1.

273

4. A select study group for special purposes here consists of married men *only* who participated at T_1, T_2 and T_3. This permits examination of a stable number of patients in terms of family illness patterns over the year. N = 259.
5. See Reference 4 above.
6. The group studied was composed of only those married couples who were interviewed at two stages. If the wife did not participate at one of the stages, data for the couple was excluded. N = 196.
7. For a description of categories, refer to Chapter 2.
8. These materials on the following pages are drawn in large part from Croog et al., 1972.

Chapter 8

PERSONALITY AND PSYCHOLOGICAL FACTORS

INTRODUCTION

Our modest purpose in this chapter is to report on some personality characteristics of the heart patients. This subject is timely and pertinent in view of the many controversies now in progress concerning the role of personality in illness. The field is marked by a variety of schools of thought and conflicting hypotheses (Friedman and Rosenman, 1974; Hellerstein et al., 1969; Ibrahim et al., 1966; Jenkins, 1971; Shekelle et al., 1970; Syme, 1975; Zohman, 1973).[1]

One persistent theme is that there are certain personality features common to cardiac patients which may be of an etiological nature. A number of critics have questioned this assumption, raising such issues as the validity and reliability of measurement of the personality construct, and the validity of conclusions derived from the research itself. In the process of rehabilitation and recovery, it is well known that personality factors may be associated with constructive coping with the illness and may serve as defense mechanisms or support systems in the "armory of resources."

In this chapter, we report some empirical evidence concerning patients' ratings on a series of their own, self-perceived personality traits at two points in time, as well as areas of change in those self-perceptions. We also consider the question of correlates of change. And in Chapter 9 we examine the additional issue of the relationship of personality self-assessment items to "outcome." These materials enlarge upon data we have presented elsewhere concerning mechanisms of denial and changes in self-image (Croog et al., 1971; Idelson et al., 1974).

The materials in this chapter are intended to serve at least two purposes. One is to portray the ways in which men who have had a heart attack see themselves. These materials help us to consider whether the post-cardiac patients share common characteristics as far as some aspects of personality are concerned. The issue is also of particular interest in view of the many hypotheses and controversies in regard to the identification of core personality patterns in the period *before* the occurrence of the heart attack. For example, the data provide a further base to explore ways in which such traits may be linked to the premorbid personality characteristics found by other investigators.

A second purpose is to focus attention on the personality characteristics of patients during an extended period of the recovery process. In this case it is possible to compare the ratings of the personality items at two points in time. In view of the minimal information now available on personality and self-perception of traits in heart patients and other types of chronically ill patients, it seems useful to review some of the empirical materials drawn from patient interviews.

Sources of Data

The primary materials reported in this chapter are based on a series of 22 self-rating items descriptive of personality traits. The series was derived from two sources, one of which was a study designed for purposes other than the investigation of coronary personality. Seventeen items were employed in scales by Burgess and Wallin for marital prediction studies, and they have subsequently been employed by various other investigators (Burgess and Wallin, 1953; Farber, 1960; Pineo, 1961). In addition, a series of five items was added to the Burgess-Wallin set by the authors. These were drawn from current conceptions about common components in the coronary personality, and they deal with such dimensions as feeling time-pressure, being hard-driving, and the exerting of effort (Jenkins, 1971).

The self-rating items were introduced into our study of heart patients as one technique for developing rapid information in a non-threatening manner on selected personality characteristics and self-perceptions. They are also used later in this volume for analyzing ways in which these individual traits might be related to various dimensions of behavior during the recovery period.

In the interviews, patients were asked to rate themselves on each trait in the series, using a five point scale ranging from "very much" to "not at all." For purposes of factor analysis, the original five category system of classification was maintained. In analysis of these data through non-parametric tests, responses were classified into three categories to ensure sufficient numbers in cells. Category 3 consisted of those responses which were "hasn't the trait at all." The categories "somewhat" and "a little" were classified into a single category and were given a code rating of 2. The responses "very much" and "considerably" were combined as a single category and were coded as 1.

The self-rating data were collected at T_2 and T_3. In the T_2 interview, patients were asked to rate themselves as to the extent each of the traits described them prior to their illness. At T_3 they were asked to rate themselves on the same traits as they described them one year after hospitalization. Of course, we cannot be sure that the patients actually viewed themselves previous to the illness in the terms that they indicated at the time of the T_2 interview. The extent to which the illness experience colored their recall and influenced their perceptions of their pre-illness state cannot be determined. As we will see later, we were able to compare some of these ratings with those made by a "normal" male population selected earlier through random sampling techniques. The data from T_2 constitute one type of retrospective assessment after an illness event and cannot be considered to represent actual pre-illness traits.

A REPORT ON FINDINGS

Self-Ratings at T_2.

In the ratings of their own pre-illness traits, men in the study population presented a picture with several apparent themes. On the whole, the heart patients portrayed themselves as men with a sense of humor, a high sense of duty, and an interest in "putting a lot of effort into things." Comparatively few reported having traits which were socially undesirable. High proportions denied being self-centered, dominating, jealous or critical of others.

Table 1. Personality Self-Assessment Ratings at T₂. Ratings by
Patients with Reference to Pre-Illness Traits.
In Percent. (N=345)

Personality Items	Ratings in Percent		
	1 (High)	2	3 (Low)
Sense of Duty	85.8	13.3	0.6
Puts Lot of Effort into Things	77.1	18.8	3.8
Sense of Humor	65.2	32.5	1.8
Easygoing	63.8	30.2	5.8
Likes Responsibility	60.6	31.6	7.5
Being in a Hurry	55.9	25.8	18.0
Ambitious	53.9	37.4	8.4
Eats Rapidly	47.8	25.5	26.4
Hard Driving	41.2	30.4	28.1
Stubborn	38.0	52.5	9.0
Nervous	28.1	46.1	25.2
Gets Angry Easily	26.4	52.9	23.2
Feelings Easily Hurt	25.5	45.5	28.4
Easily Excited	25.5	40.9	33.0
Likes Organizations	17.1	37.1	45.5
Critical of Others	14.8	41.4	43.5
Moody	13.0	46.7	39.7
Easily Depressed	12.8	39.4	47.2
Dominating	12.2	35.1	51.6
Shy	10.7	42.9	46.1
Self-Centered	6.7	40.3	51.9
Jealous	4.9	18.6	75.9

1 (High) = Very much or considerably; 2 = Somewhat or a little;
3 (Low) = Not at all

In view of the stereotyped portrayal of the heart patient as ambitious, restless and putting effort into things, it is interesting to note that to a considerable extent these patients portray themselves in these terms. Devotion to duty, ambition, being in a hurry, liking responsibility are all reported with substantial representation in categories 1 and 2. These distributions do not, of course, indicate anything about the relationship of personality traits to etiology.

To some extent, of course, these traits fit the image of the American male as he is sometimes portrayed in folklore: hard-working, ambitious, hard-driving, yet at the same time easygoing or casual and with a good sense of humor. In fact, given the currency of stereotypes, it is surprising that six men in the group were bold enough to describe themselves as not having a sense of humor! Like the image in folklore and in real life, there are inconsistencies in this self-portrayal picture.

An exploration was carried out to determine whether there were significant statistical associations between self-rating items and major social identity variables of Type 1: age, educational level, occupational level and social class. This was done on the possibility that these variables exerted influence upon the distribution of ratings. Our procedures turned up no convincing evidence that age was related to personality self-assessment in this study group.[2]

In regard to educational level, too, there were virtually no gamma scores in which the accompanying chi-square level was significant, and which met minimal criteria for calculation (i.e. having sufficient numbers in cells). The main finding was in regard to "critical of others."[3] The relationship was not linear. Given the fact that this, the strongest finding, is not a very powerful result, we may conclude that the remaining, even weaker set of associations show little valid evidence of association between educational level and personality self-ratings at T_2. Hence, in the absence of promising evidence of association with personality items, no controls for age, education, occupation and social class were employed in subsequent analysis of the items.

Response Patterns in Self-Ratings: A Factor Analysis

Are there underlying clusters of traits which may help us to understand how the personality ratings are interrelated within the study population? In the case of the present study, we have used factor analysis as a means of condensing the personality rating items and eliciting some of the possible underlying constructs.[4] It is important to note that the loadings and factors are not a function of the amounts of various traits which the subjects possess. Instead, they reflect the interrelationships between the ratings on personality items.

Factor analysis was carried out for the study population as a whole at T_2 and without use of control variables. The factor analysis of the 22 personality self-rating items yielded seven factors which, taken together, account for 60.5 percent of the total variance.

Factor 1, as can be seen, accounts for 20 percent of the total variance. Its highest loadings occur in regard to such traits as "nervous," "feelings easily hurt," and "easily excited." On the basis of the general pattern, we have called this factor "emotional reactivity," a reflection of high sensitivity and lability, which the individual items seem to represent.

The clustering of traits in Factor 2, may be labeled "dominance-narcissism." It accounts for 12 percent of the variance. Here there is a pattern of characteristics which may go along with traits of aggressiveness and competitiveness. The best measures of this factor are such traits as "dominating," "critical of others," "self-

Table 2. Factor Analysis of Personality Self-Rating Items.
Rotated Factor Loadings. Product at T_2 (N=340).*

Factor 1. Emotional Reactivity (20.3%)		Factor 2. Dominance-Narcissism (11.6%)	
Nervous	.732	Dominating	.758
Feelings hurt	.698	Critical of others	.746
Easily excited	.694	Self-centered	.552
Easily depressed	.664	Stubborn	.518
Easily angered	.644	Easygoing	-.434
Moody	.628	Easily angered	.348
In a hurry	.332	Hard-driving	.306

Factor 3. Ambition (6.6%)		Factor 4. View of Competition (6.3%)	
Ambitious	.736	Jealous	.679
Puts in effort	.728	Likes organizations	.666
Responsibility	.710	Easygoing	.352
Sense of duty	.509		
Hard-driving	.472		

Factor 5. Sensitivity (5.8%)		Factor 6. Pressured Activity (5.2%)	
Shy	.805	Eats rapidly	.832
Self-centered	.451	In a hurry	.681
Easily depressed	.330	Hard-driving	.541
		Nervous	.312

Factor 7. Extroverted-Conscientious (4.7%)	
Sense of humor	.826
Sense of duty	.534
Easygoing	.316

* The numbers in parentheses after each of the factors represent the percentage of variance accounted for by each factor.

centered," and "stubborn."

Factor 3 has its highest loadings on "being ambitious," "putting a lot of effort into things," and "likes responsibility." This factor accounts for seven percent of the variance. Although, as we have noted, the factor does not represent the amount and direction of the trait in the population, its internal structure brings to mind one of the most common characterizations in the literature about heart patients: It may be labeled "Ambition."

With Factor 3 we move to consideration of those factors which explain relatively small proportions of the variance. In fact, as can be seen, the remainder are not very different from Factor 3 in percentage of variance accounted for. Among the remainder, perhaps the sixth factor, "pressured activity," is most interesting. Its high loadings are on "being in a hurry," "eating rapidly," and "being hard-driving." Without reference to amount or direction of loadings, these areas are reminiscent of the Friedman-Rosenman characterization of the coronary-prone behavior pattern and the sense of time urgency (Friedman and Rosenman, 1974). This factor, however, accounts for only five percent of the variance.

In sum, the findings present a condensed view of the internal patterns of the personality self-rating responses. Factor 1 represents a cluster of interrelated variables reflecting anxiety and emotional instability. The second factor is measured by a series of core traits indicative of the aggressive, dominating, egocentric, volatile type of personality orientation.

In connection with these emergent factors in the self-rating data, there are several issues which affect interpretation. Although the men were asked to rate themselves as they were before their recent infarction, some of these factors may be explained in terms of immediate reactions to the heart attack or to the interview situation. As with any retrospective data, the influence of the heart attack may have had an effect on the derived factors.

Since it was not feasible to use a control group in this particular study, we must acknowledge that "healthy men" of the same social background might develop the same factor structure. It is not possible to assess the degree to which the factors found here may simply be a product of male self-image in an American urban setting, as well as a function of the self-perception items included.

The possibility that the factors are merely describing common American traits rather than special characteristics of heart patients is clearly one which deserves further careful scrutiny. Systematic employment of control groups drawn from normal populations will aid considerably in resolving this question. In the interim, however, some available data from the Framingham Heart Study and from our own data on the wives of the heart patients may provide some useful clues.

The Heart Patients and a Normal Population: Comparisons with the Framingham Heart Study Population

As noted earlier, there is no implication concerning etiology in relation to these data. In the absence of a control group, it is impossible to state that these characteristics as reported distinguish the heart patients from other men in the so-called "normal" population. Some available materials from another independent study, however, present some unusual opportunities for comparisons between personality self-ratings. These give some indications as to how these perceptions by the heart patients differ from those of men in an adjacent geographic area and within similar age categories.

During the period of data collection for this report, one of the authors (Levine) collaborated with Norman A. Scotch in a study of the role of social and psychological stress in the etiology of heart disease. This research was carried out in conjunction with the Framingham Heart Study, one of the best known longitudinal studies of illness etiology (Gordon et al., 1971).

As part of the continuing monitoring and data collection processes of the Framingham Heart Study, male and female participants were provided with a free physical examination at two year intervals over two decades. During the course of these examinations, various types of tests and data collection were carried out. In the eighth and ninth examinations, as part of the Levine-Scotch inquiry, respondents were also interviewed concerning a series of life stresses.

The Framingham study population was a "normal" cohort originally, and it was not selected on the basis of coronary disease. It was not a representative sample at the time of the collection of the Scotch-Levine data, however, for attrition of the original population over time had occurred. Nevertheless, within these limitations it is useful for comparative purposes here.

In the course of their interviews at Framingham, respondents were asked to make self-ratings on a series of items concerning personality traits. In addition, they were asked to respond to a series of questions pertaining to level of perceived stress.[5] Some comparison of these data with materials from the study population is possible, insofar as there was considerable communality between our heart patient group and the Framingham study population in the listing of personality rating items. Complete comparison of responses is not possible, however, since our study and the Framingham one used somewhat differing personality rating scales. In the present study, as has been indicated, participants were asked how well the term described them. The five response categories were "very much," "considerably," "somewhat," "a little," and "not at all." This follows the usage in the original Burgess and Wallin instrument (Burgess and Wallin, 1953). In the Framingham research, however, the four categories were "very well," "fairly well," "somewhat," and "not at all."

Although the full range of data from the two studies cannot be compared, it is of interest to examine the extreme categories where respondents chose to place themselves. In the case of Reeder and Levine-Scotch questions, no problems of phrasing comparability are present, since the exact wording was used in the two studies.

The distributions of responses are reported in Table 3. In this table the age groups "less than 55" and "55-65" years are reported. Two things should be noted. We have not subdivided the heart patient population into age categories, but rather, we present data on the total group. This procedure has been followed inasmuch as no variation was previously found in personality self-rating items in terms of age. Second, as will be seen in Table 3, there is minimal variation by age in the self-rating items in the Framingham group. Though the age range in the heart patient population does not extend beyond 60, we include the broader age group 55-65 for Framingham. Since there is minimal variation between the age groups of Framingham and since the differences with the heart patient group are minor, it was not deemed necessary to reclassify in order to report completely comparable age categories in the table.

The left segment of Table 3 shows a comparison of the heart patient responses on "very much" with the highest rating for the Framingham respondents, "very well." The right segment shows the proportion in both populations who responded "not at all." In both populations, as can be seen, the proportions are similar. On the Chi-square statistical test, there are no significant differences between groups.

Thus, it appears that as compared with men from the general population in a community, the heart patient population does not differ markedly in terms of the crude percentages reported here. It should be pointed out that a minority of subjects in the Framingham population had been coronary cases, others were developing symptoms but were pre-clinical, and we may

Table 3. Heart Patient Population and Framingham Study Population. Responses on Personality Self-Rating Items. In Percent. By Age Groups. Males Only.

	Highest Rating (Describes me "very well" or "very much")			Lowest Rating (Describes me "not at all")		
	Heart Patients 30-60 (N=345)	Framingham Group 54 and Under (N=519)	Framingham Group 55-65 (N=409)	Heart Patients 30-60 (N=345)	Framingham Group 54 and Under (N=519)	Framingham Group 55-65 (N=408)
Easygoing	37.2	37.3	40.4	5.3	2.1	2.4
Sense of Humor	36.0	43.4	49.2	1.7	.7	–
Hard Driving and Competitive*	26.5	14.5	12.1	28.0	33.5	43.5
Gets Angry Easily	15.4	12.7	11.7	23.4	26.2	30.4
Feelings Easily Hurt	14.8	12.0	14.0	28.1	22.4	25.4
Easily Excited	13.1	14.0	14.2	33.1	26.4	30.4
Easily Depressed	6.7	5.7	6.1	47.1	35.8	40.7
Bossy or Dominating*	6.4	5.4	5.0	51.5	47.6	49.2

* Terms employed in Framingham study questionnaire. In Heart Patient study, the terms "Dominating" and "Hard Driving" were used, rather than "Bossy or Dominating" or "Hard Driving and Competitive." Although the items are not directly comparable, data are presented here for descriptive purposes.

hypothesize that still others were precoronary (i.e., they would eventually develop symptoms but as yet manifested no signs). If there is such a clinical phenomenon as a "coronary personality," the presence of these men with symptoms and those in pre-symptom condition would serve to reduce differences between the Framingham study group and those in the heart patient population. Empirical resolution of this issue was not within the resources or aims of the present study, and we

Table 4. Heart Patient Population and Framingham Study
Population. Responses on Work Tension and Stress
Questions.* In Percent. Males Only.

"Yes" Response Only	Heart Patients 30-60** (N=345)	Framingham Group 30-65 (N=927)
Work stays with me after hours	49.6	38.0
Often feel pressed for time	44.6	40.6
Work affects my digestion, sleep, health	33.3	15.2
Feeling of dissatisfaction with work	33.0	34.4

*The following items, developed by researchers in the Midtown Manhattan Study, were asked of heart patients at T_2 as follows: "Now we are interested in how you generally felt at the end of an average day in your regular line of work before you became sick.
  A. Did you often have a feeling of dissatisfaction with your work?
  B. Did your work often affect your digestion or sleep, or upset your health in any way?
  C. Did your work often stay with you so that you were thinking about it after working hours?
  D. Did you often feel pressed for time?

Respondents in the Framingham study group were asked the same questions, except that they were requested to answer as of the time current to the interview.

**Data are not presented by age category for reasons explained in the text in relation to Table 3.

report here solely on the comparisons which were actually made.

On another set of questions, other types of comparisons are possible. Responses to a series of questions regarding work and stress relating to personality traits are reported in Tables 4 and 5, comparing the heart study and Framingham research populations. As may be seen, similar proportions report feelings of dissatisfaction with their work. Somewhat higher proportions of heart patients report ruminating on their work after hours. The most marked differences occur in response to the question regarding perception of work as affecting health or digestion.

Further, as the data in Table 5 indicate, higher proportions of the heart patients responded that before their heart attack they experienced a great amount of strain in connection with their daily activities. Considerably higher proportions also reported themselves as usually tense and nervous.

These additional data serve further to differentiate the heart patient group from that of a so-called "normal" population. It should be emphasized that the responses may simply reflect screened perceptions and post-heart attack explanations—i.e., that work stress and working too hard caused the illness. In any case, regardless of etiological implications, it would appear that higher proportions in the heart patient group portray themselves through these questions as tense and nervous and as living under stress.

The Wives of the Heart Patients

Another facet to the issue of self-image of heart patients as compared with other populations is seen in data which we collected from the wives of the heart patient population. As noted earlier in this volume, the wives of

Table 5. Nervous Strain and Feelings of Tension. Heart Patient Population and Framingham Study Group. In Percent. Males Only. By Age Groups*

	Response Category					*N*
	Very Well	*Fairly Well*	*Not Very Well*	*Not At All*	*No Response, Don't Know*	
High nervous strain in daily activities						
Heart patients 30-60	23.4	32.5	16.8	26.7	.6	345
Framingham men** 30-54	10.0	25.2	23.1	35.5	6.2	519
55-65	8.1	26.4	17.0	41.0	7.5	408
Unusually tense and nervous						
Heart patients 30-60	24.1	24.1	22.0	29.3	.5	345
Framingham men 30-54	5.0	13.7	26.4	48.7	6.2	519
55-65	4.2	13.4	21.5	53.2	7.7	408

* The following items, developed by Leo G. Reeder were asked of heart patients at T_2 in regard to how they felt at the end of an average day before they became sick:

A. There was a great deal of nervous strain connected with my daily activities.

B. In general, I was unusually tense and nervous.

** Respondents in the Framingham study group were asked to report as of the time current to the interview.

patients were interviewed at the T_2 and the T_3 stages. At those times, instruments were used similar to those employed for the men. Thus, at T_2 we collected information from the wives in regard to their own self-perceptions of personality traits, using the same format as for the men. These and additional materials on wives are being reported in other publications (Croog and Fitzgerald, 1978).

The study population of wives at T_2 consisted of

283 participants. One feature of the personality self-descriptions of this group at T_2 was their general similarity to the husband population in patterns of ratings (Croog et al., 1976). On each item, when the pattern of husband populations and wife populations was compared, there were no significant differences. In addition, a factor analysis produced similar patterns of factors.

These results were *not* due to the fact that "like married like," i.e., that ambitious, time-urgent men tended to marry women who were similar. In fact, there was little correlation between self-image patterns on individual traits when husband-wife pairs were examined. Rather, the explanation may derive from the possibility that in this age group the two separate populations may really be mirroring the larger general population. It may be hypothesized that some of the phenomena are due to a common set of personality themes or socially determined styles of self-description characteristic more of the population in general than of heart patients in particular. How this fits reality can best be tested through empirical research with closer, more directed assessment of these themes in male and female American populations.

Continuities and Change in Self-Ratings

Given this picture of self-ratings at T_2, what was the stability of these self-assessments over time? One issue associated with this question centers on the relationship of the illness experience to the persistence of personality traits. There are several research dimensions to this issue. One involves ascertaining the relative rankings according to degree of stability or change over time. In other words, within the total series, which ratings change more than others, and with which aspects of personality are the patterns of change concerned?

A second matter for investigation relates to the direction of change. Here we are concerned with whether the move is in the direction of such traits as volatility, anxiety, and other indicators of personal distress, or in the direction of integration, stability and control.

The third matter for inquiry is the relationship of the illness experience to change and stability. In this context, since all the men were initially ill with the same ailment, the question devolves into the relationship of severity and recurrence over the year with changes in self-perception.

There are, of course, numerous variables which may explain change in self-ratings over time. Here we are concerned, however, only with the question of the illness experience and the change in personality self-reassessment. In this exploratory work, regardless of positive or negative findings, the contribution of additional underlying variables cannot be ruled out. It seems desirable, however, to report some of the apparent trends, which may provide a base-point for future studies.

Table 6 presents data on stability of self-ratings within the population of patients who participated in interviews at both the T_2 and T_3 stages. These materials are reported as the percentage of men who rated themselves in the same category at T_3 as they did at T_2. As may be seen, for some items such as sense of humor, sense of duty, and jealousy, 73 percent and over described themselves in the same terms. At the other end of the scale, approximately half of those who initially described themselves as hard-driving, easily angered, and easily excited continued to rate themselves in the same way one year afterwards. In reviewing the data from the obverse standpoint, the findings indicate that from one-fifth to one-half of the men who remained in the study altered their self-ratings over time.

The direction of change for each item is shown in

Table 6. Stability in Personality Self-Ratings from T_2 to T_3.
Three Point Scale*

Personality Items At T_2	Stability Base N = Total Subjects Who Gave Ratings**	Ratings Remaining Stable From T_2 to T_3 In Percent of Base N
Sense of Duty	291	81.1
Sense of Humor	292	73.6
Jealous	290	73.4
Puts a Lot of Effort Into Things	291	68.7
Likes Organizations	292	67.1
Likes Responsibility	289	66.1
Stubborn	290	65.9
Self-Centered	289	64.4
Shy	291	63.2
Easygoing	292	63.0
Dominating	290	62.8
Eats Rapidly	292	62.3
Easily Depressed	290	61.4
Ambitious	292	60.0
Moody	287	59.6
Critical of Others	292	59.2
In A Hurry	292	57.2
Feelings Easily Hurt	290	57.2
Easily Excited	290	55.5
Nervous	287	55.0
Gets Angry Easily	290	50.0
Hard Driving	291	48.4

* For purposes of this Table, the initial five categories were condensed as follows: 1 = High; 2 = Medium; 3 = Low. N includes respondents in all three categories whose rating remained stable.

** Variation in size of N on items is due to occurrence of non-response or indecision by respondent.

Table 7. Here the population of changers is presented, considering only those with potential for movement upward or downward. Thus, the base is not the total population, but rather the total number in the categories available for change. Those with the potential for *increase* were in two categories: "not at all," and "somewhat." Hence the proportion of those who changed is computed using the ratio of changers in relation to the total in the two categories. Similarly, the potential group for movement *downward* includes those in the "very much" and the "somewhat" categories. These are used as the base number for computing the movement downward. This procedure means that the category "somewhat" is used twice for computation of change, since it is in the middle of the classification. It also means that the percentages for change cannot be added together as "changers" since they overlap in sharing part of the same base. It is also inappropriate to consider the total changers from Table 7 in summing up in combination with the "stables" in Table 6. This system of calculation for the direction of change, however, has the advantage of considering only the men with potential for change as part of the computation. While other systems may attain similar results eventually, this method presents immediate evidence on the issue.

The percentages in Table 7 show several interesting features. On most items, the net difference in percentages of items of change was relatively low. Among men for whom there was potential for change, on only several items was there any massive indication of movement upward or downward. Relatively high proportions in the categories with potential for change upward reported high net change in the direction of "sense of duty," "hard-driving," and "easygoing." Highest net decrease was on such items as "jealous," and "self-centered." These changes might perhaps be interpreted as being in

Table 7. Change in Personality Self-Ratings from T_2 to T_3. By Direction of Change. Three Point Scale

Personality Self-Rating Items	Increase*		Decrease*	
	Base N = N Potential for Increase from T_2 to T_3; N = Low (3) and Medium (2)	Increase In Percent	Base N = N Potential for Decrease from T_2 to T_3; N = Medium (2) and High (1)	Decrease In Percent
Sense of Humor	97	27.8	288	17.4
Sense of Duty	40	67.5	289	9.7
Stubborn	177	28.8	264	18.2
Gets Angry Easily	213	36.2	223	30.5
Feelings Easily Hurt	218	23.4	208	35.1
Nervous	207	35.7	210	26.2
Easygoing	96	41.7	277	24.5
Moody	246	22.8	176	34.1
Jealous	274	12.0	68	64.7
Likes Responsibility	110	38.2	271	20.7
Dominating	256	21.1	141	38.3
Critical	248	21.8	171	38.0
Easily Excited	216	34.7	191	28.3

Personality Self-Rating Items	Increase*		Decrease*	
	Base N = N Potential for Increase from T_2 to T_3; N = Low (3) and Medium (2)	Increase In Percent	Base N = N Potential for Decrease from T_2 to T_3; N = Medium (2) and High (1)	Decrease In Percent
Shy	259	27.8	159	22.0
Likes Organizations	239	18.8	160	31.9
Easily Depressed	153	35.3	152	38.2
Self-Centered	271	16.2	136	43.4
In A Hurry	130	27.8	236	37.7
Ambitious	136	33.1	267	27.0
Eats Rapidly	151	23.2	216	34.7
Hard Driving	174	60.3	209	21.5
Puts Lot of Effort Into Things	67	38.8	281	23.1

* This table on change contains information drawn only from categories with potential for showing change. For example, data in base N for "Increase" column contain total number of responses for "Not at All" and "Some" categories and data from "Very much" is omitted. Movement higher from "Very much" category is not possible, and hence it would be inappropriate to include it as part of the base. Similarly, in computation of proportions moving downward in ratings, the "Not at all" category is excluded from the base N. Here again, movement downward beyond "Not at all" is not possible, so these data are omitted. A three-point scale is employed (See note at bottom of Table 6).

the "socially approved" direction.

Most notable is the lack of consistent pattern of net movement in one direction for any set of items. Among those who changed in their ratings on emotional volatility, such as angering easily, easily excited, and easily depressed, the proportion reporting an increase was similar to that reporting a decrease. Moreover, inconsistencies come through with movement both in the direction of being "easygoing" and being "hard-driving." Since these items are self-assessments, the issue of validity of the ratings is only one aspect of the problem of interpretation. These data may indicate a number of other phenomena, such as actual changes in self-perceptions, the operation of denial or self-aggrandizement in ratings or variation in level of cooperation in the interview. Another possible source of influence is the level of severity of illness, and this matter is discussed in the next section.

Change in Ratings and Severity of Illness

The final question for consideration here is the relation between level of illness and changes in personal self-ratings. In order to carry out this analysis, three groups of patients were compared: (a) those who were rehospitalized one or more times during the 11 months following initial discharge from hospital, (b) those who were not rehospitalized but were described by their physicians as having developed significant additional illness during the year, and (c) those who were neither rehospitalized nor described by their physicians in ways similar to those in category b. (Discussion of classification of the three groups is provided in Chapter 2.)

The nature of the distributions within each of the three categories presents some limitations on the analysis. In some instances, there are insufficient numbers in cells to justify reporting conclusions. This problem is compounded by several factors: distribution of the total population into illness levels, skewed distributions in ratings on self-description items, and variations in the numbers of persons who changed in their ratings.

In the analysis three separate types of tabulations were carried out. Each of the sets of ratings was examined separately, using the "not at all," "somewhat," and "very much" categories as the three separate spheres. Within each one, cross tabulations were performed, comparing T_2 with T_3 responses, and controlling for illness severity level. Analysis of these distributions revealed no significant differences by levels of illness severity in regard to changes in reported self-perceptions.

Nevertheless, some interpretations are suggested by this finding. One is that personality self-ratings are not significantly altered by circumstances such as illness. To put it another way, the fact that a man previously considered himself as volatile, hard-driving, or nervous may not be altered simply by the fact of illness. It is a common theme among the patients that they were under strain, that they were nervous and hard-working. Further, it is commonly believed among heart patients (and doctors have advised) that it is desirable to slow down, take things easier, avoid strain and emotional upset in order to minimize risk of future heart attacks. In the case of these data, however, there is no evidence that the men who were severely ill were most likely to change in their views of themselves.

It is possible, of course, that the men did change in their personalities but that they simply did not perceive themselves as having changed. We have no data with which to support or deny this, however.

Another aspect of personality self-ratings, aside from the issue of change, is their relationship to outcome or status at one year. This question is reviewed as part of the larger appraisal of outcome in Chapter 9.

Personality Self-Ratings and the Denial Mechanism: Empirical Observations

It has long been observed by clinicians that the denial response is a common phenomenon in cardiac patients during the first stages after their heart attack (Dunbar, 1948, 1954; Hackett and Weisman, 1969). The manifestations of denial and its persistence over time have rarely been subjected to empirical study with sizeable populations of patients, however. In our research on the heart patient population, several principal findings emerged which merit brief review. They are reported in more detail in another publication (Croog et al., 1971).

At T_1, patients were asked, "From what you know about your own illness, do you think you have had a heart attack?" Twenty percent of respondents expressed denial at that time. Three aspects of the denial response then were further explored: social and psychological correlates, generalization of the denial response to other areas of the patients' lives, and the continuity of denial over time. Of interest here is the possible relationship between personality self-ratings and the denial response.

Considering ratings on individual personality trait items at T_2 and T_3, no meaningful and statistically significant differences were found between deniers and non-deniers. When the personality items were classified for analytic purposes as "negative" and "non-negative," deniers tended to disavow possessing unfavorable traits.[6] Deniers reported more depression than non-deniers, but indicated less severity of depression when it was present. They also generalized denial to other areas of their lives, disavowing, for example, that they had significant problems. In general, considering the possible persistence of

the denial mechanism over the course of the year, those
who denied initially tended to minimize the impact of
the illness upon their lives.

SUMMARY

In this chapter we have reported on two sets of self-ratings of personality traits, as presented by patients at T_2
and T_3 interviews. No associations were found between
these ratings and age, educational and occupational level.
Hence, we have considered the patient population as a
whole, without employing controls for these variables.

According to their own description, the patients in
highest proportions described themselves as having a
sense of duty, liking responsibility, putting a lot of effort
into things. Half rated themselves as "very much" or
"considerably" in a hurry, "ambitious," and "eating
rapidly." These ratings, recorded one month after discharge from hospital, were made by patients in response
to a request that they characterize how they were before
the illness.

Further examination of ratings at T_2 was carried
out through factor analysis. Here a set of factors
emerged which indicated the internal dimensions of
emotionality, volatility, ambition, narcissism-dominance,
among others. The possibility was suggested that results
were in part influenced by the fact of illness.

Opportunity for comparison of some of these
responses with those from a group of men from a "normal" population arose with the availability of data from
the Framingham Heart Study. On those items for which
limited comparisons could be made after dichotomizing,
there was marked similarity in ratings. Main areas in
which the heart patients differed from the Framingham
group was in their assessments of themselves as nervous

and under strain at work. Aside from the stress items, however, there were no differences between the self-ratings of the two groups when ratings were statistically adjusted to permit analysis. Moreover, the heart patients' assessments of their own personality traits did not differ significantly from the assessments reported by their wives.

On each rating, from half to four-fifths of the men at T_3 had given the same response at T_2. Among those who changed their responses, there were mixed findings which were inconclusive, as far as direction upward or downward was concerned. Level of severity of illness during the year was not found to be related to change in self-perception. Whether they changed or not in their self-perception, the illness experience did not seem to be related to the stability or change in rating.

NOTES

1. For additional references covering personality and heart disease, see: Caffrey, 1961; Caffrey, 1967; Cleveland and Johnson, 1962; Doyle, 1966; Cady et al., 1961; Friedman et al., 1968; Ibrahim et al., 1967; Jenkins et al., 1974; Keith et al., 1965; Master, 1960; Medalle et al., 1973; Miles et al., 1954; Minc et al., 1963; Mordkoff and Parsons, 1967; Ostfeld et al., 1964; Pearson and Joseph, 1963; Rosenman et al., 1970; Russek and Zohman, 1958; Sprague, 1958; Wardwell et al., 1963; Weiss et al., 1957.
2. Of the series of items, the highest gamma score was .27, indicating a relationship between age and being jealous. However, there were small numbers in those cells indicating some degree of jealousy. Though the Chi-square findings show significance, this must be set aside since criteria were not met in regard to numbers in cells.
3. Chi-square = 25.45, df = 4, p < .001; gamma = .30.
4. Factor analysis was carried out through the use of the SPSS Program on the UNIVAC 1106. The standard principal components factor analysis was computed for the total study population of 345 respondents and for 22 individual items. The criteria for extracting roots were as follows: maximum number of factors = 8.0. Minimum latent root = 1.00. The minimum percent of communality was set at 10.00. Rotation by variables was carried out through the Orthogonal Varimax technique. Through these

techniques, 6 factors were produced by the computer with loadings ranging from .731 to −.649. In this presentation only traits
which have loadings greater than an absolute value of .30 are recorded as important in contributing to the factors.

The factor analysis method was chosen, insofar as it constitutes a
useful means for classifying and condensing phenomena into
underlying sets of variables. It aids in the conceptual simplifica-
tion of the items into a more manageable framework. Though
there are difficulties in the interpretation of factors in this procedure, the technique helps to limit the possibilities of investigator
bias. It is evident that a purely mathematical inspection of
underlying test structure provides a guide for further conceptual
work. For additional information, see: R. Cattell, 1952; Kerlinger,
1964 and Nunnally, 1967.

5. The indices of perceived stress are drawn from the Life History
   Questionnaire used for a study of life stress and heart disease,
   Framingham Heart Study, and from questions developed by Leo
   G. Reeder at the University of California, Los Angeles. The
   question, "Did your work often affect your digestion or sleep, or
   upset your health in any way?" is adapted from one employed in
   the Midtown Manhattan Study. See Langner and Michael, 1963,
   p. 313. For additional information, see J.M. Chapman et al.,
   1966; M. Schar et al., 1973; and Reeder et al., 1973.

6. "Negative" traits were as follows: feelings easily hurt, gets angry
   easily, nervous or irritable, being in a hurry, eating rapidly, easily
   depressed, stubborn, self-centered, easily excited, moody, critical
   of others, jealous, being hard driving, shy, and dominating or
   bossy. "Non-negative" traits were: being ambitious, sense of
   humor, likes organizations, sense of duty, easy going, putting a
   lot of effort into things, and likes responsibility.

Chapter 9

THE PATIENTS AT ONE YEAR: A REVIEW OF STATUSES AND ASSOCIATED VARIABLES

INTRODUCTION

Status at One Year and Antecedent Variables

How were the men faring one year after their first myocardial infarction? The issue of "outcome" in prospective studies of this sort is one which commonly presents numerous problems of conceptualization, measurement, and value judgments. The problem may be formulated, for example, in terms of "level of adjustment" or "degree of adaptation" at the end of a given period. Yet what constitutes "adjustment" or "adaptation" obviously depends upon a range of factors, such as pre-illness condition, valuation of pre-illness adjustment, and criteria for measuring "adjustment" at the end of the study year in terms of objective and subjective factors.

Hence, as we indicated in Chapter 1, our approach

here is to move away as much as possible from using
evaluative criteria, relying primarily instead on a series
of "snapshots" at a point in time, one year after the
heart attack. These center on indices of status, each of
which deals with a differing dimension in the life of the
patient. As we shall see, the measures vary from the
relatively objective, such as work status, to the more
highly subjective, those involving, for example, patients'
feelings about the meaning of their lives and their
degree of satisfaction with it. Further, rather than a
single additive and simplistic measure, we have chosen to
look at a series of key areas, each dealing with a major
aspect of the lives of the patients—work, activity,
psychological state, and view of life, and other areas as
described in the following pages. Our hope is that with a
population so varied and complex as is our study population, consideration of the separate parts will add up to
more than a simple sum of the whole.

   Drawing upon pre-illness and early illness information, what social and psychological factors were
associated with the status of the men in the study population one year after their heart attack? In this chapter
we first report data on several selected indicators of
status or condition at T_3. We then turn to an exploratory examination of the possible association of items in a
series of antecedent variables with the year-end status
indicators.

   While the empirical exploration of possible associations of variables with status at one year has been the
primary effort, it has been guided by a continuing
theme. The issue of armory of resources has constituted
one touchstone as a frame of reference. As we indicated
in the first chapter, a purpose of this study has been to
learn whether men with supports in major areas of their
lives, those with particular social and psychological
resources, do better than those who lack such resources

or who possess them in lesser degrees. In this chapter we are asking whether men who are socially integrated do better than those who are less integrated. The research questions guiding the selection of items have been based on a set of assumptions concerning the importance of family, work situation, religious orientation, and social participation as elements in the patient's "armory of resources." Is status at the end of the year related to pre-illness evidence of emotional support in marriage, high satisfaction and minimal stress at work, support as indicated by participation in the religious institution, and integration in informal social groups?

We have assumed that a relatively high level of physical activity and a feeling of optimism before the illness may also be related to patient status at the end of the year.

Status or Condition at One Year in Areas of Life Functioning

As indices of the illness-related statuses of the patients at T_3, two series of variables were selected. For purposes of this analysis, these are classified as primary and secondary illness-outcome variables.

In this selection and classification, a main purpose has been to touch upon several dimensions of the life and emotions of the patients as they relate to the illness, keeping as close to the empirical data as possible. Hence we have relied upon first-order data from patients and their physicians, instead of developing these further into composite indices. This method also permits the separate examination of each variable as part of the total situational configuration of the patients.

PRIMARY INDICES.   Three primary variables are used, each drawn from a differing source. These are (1) the physician's clinical assessment of the patients at T_3 in terms of their functional capacity and activity level, (2) the reported perceptions by patients at T_3 in regard to their own progress, and (3) the work status of the patients at T_3.

The third variable, it will be recalled, was employed as a follow-up measure in the chapter on work. There it was used in its most obvious meaning, as a simple indicator of employment history. This same variable, however, can also serve a larger purpose. The work status of the patient is also one possible indicator of the patient's health condition. It is, of course, not an infallible indicator of adjustment or level of health. Obviously, sick patients may be employed full-time, and for many reasons well persons may not be employed. Given the importance of work as a life orientation for men in this age group, we employ this variable simply to indicate status in regard to this major life activity one year after hospital admission. It has the advantage over other measures in that it is not based upon reported perceptions or judgments of either patient or doctor but upon objective measures.

SECONDARY INDICES. The secondary variables of status at T_3 are more focused than the three primary variables. These deal with patient assessments of specific aspects of physical health, emotional status and life circumstances. They include the following:

1. *Life returned to normal.* This is based upon responses to the question, "Now that about a year has passed since you first became ill, do you feel that life has returned to normal?"
2. *Feelings of depression or discouragement.* This is based upon the responses to, "After an illness many patients feel discouraged or depressed. Do you ever feel discouraged or depressed over your illness?"
3. *Satisfaction with way of life.* This item is furnished

by answers to the question, "On the whole, how satisfied are you with your way of life today?"

4. *Index of symptoms.* This item refers to the symptoms associated with heart disease and other illness reported by the patient as having been present during the month previous to the T_3 interview. The items about which patients were questioned were: getting tired easily, chest pain, breathlessness, "feeling heart is pounding or skipping a beat," swelling of feet or ankles, sleeplessness, restlessness or nervousness, or other symptoms as specified by the patient. Reports of the number of these symptoms during the month previous to the interview were coded as follows: none; one or two = low; three to seven or more = high. In some cases, the "none" and "low" categories were combined in order to satisfy Chi-square test criteria regarding minimum cell size. The latter method of coding was used in Tables 2, 4, and 5.

5. *Perceived gains of illness.* This item is based on answers to the following question: "Despite all the problems and worries which your illness has involved, do you see any possible gains or advantages coming out of this experience?"

6. *Maintenance of pre-illness activity level.* This index question derives from information provided by the patient regarding his own perceptions of change. The patient was asked to consider his current level of activity in relation to his pre-illness level. He was then asked, "Would you say you are more active, as active, or less active than you were before?" Most patients reported change in their level of activity, with 73 percent of the total indicating less activity than before. Of the others, 20 percent remained the same and seven

percent reported they were more active than before. In the computation of tests of association, our main interest was in those patients who declined in activity level. To maximize numbers of cells, the decreasers were compared with "other," i.e., those who remained the same and those who increased.

These secondary variables thus each deal with physical symptoms experienced and feelings about satisfaction with life. There are, of course, numerous other variables which might serve as status indicator items at T_3, such as marital happiness or social participation. The chosen primary and secondary indices, however, are considered insofar as they reflect a variety of key aspects of the patients' outcome experience, given the resources of this project. It should be noted, furthermore, that status index variables at T_3 pertaining to work, marriage, personality, and life course have already been reported throughout the text.

STATUS OF PATIENTS AT ONE YEAR: A REVIEW OF FINDINGS

I. The Primary Index Variables

DISTRIBUTIONS AND RELATIONSHIPS. At one year after the first hospital admission, the three primary indices of patient status show a consistent pattern among those who survived and participated at the third state. As may be seen in the first column in Table 1, three-fourths of the patients in the study population were employed on a full-time basis. More than half the patients at T_3 were rated by their physicians as able to return to full activity, and only a minor proportion were labeled as having def-

inite limitations. The view by patients of their own
progress reflected a relatively favorable appraisal.
One-third indicated that they were doing better than
they had expected, and only 15 percent reported they
were doing worse than they expected.

Table 1.   Primary Index Variables.   Status at T_3.
Total Population and by Rehospitalization.

Primary Index Variables at T_3	Total Population†	Rehospitalized	Not Rehospitalized
Work Status			
Full-time	76.4	56.2[a]	82.0
Part-time	7.2	9.4	6.6
Unemployed	16.4	34.4	11.4
Total Percent	100.0	100.0	100.0
Total N	292	64	228
Physician Rating*			
1. (High)	62.4	39.6[a]	68.2
2. (Medium)	25.4	29.1	24.4
3. (Low)	12.2	31.3	7.4
Total Percent	100.0	100.0	100.0
Total N	237	48	189
Patient Assessment			
1. Better than expected	36.6	33.3[b]	37.6
2. As well as expected	47.7	39.7	50.0
3. Not as well as expected	15.7	27.0	12.4
Total Percent	100.0	100.0	100.0
Total N	281	63	218

[a],[b] On Chi-square test comparing the rehospitalized with the non-rehospitalized group, a = $p<.01$, b = $p<.05$.

* Physician ratings, as indicated elsewhere in text were as follows:
1 = Return to full activity, no significant impairment
2 = Return to full activity but with significant modifications
3 = Definite residual limitations on work and other activities

† Numbers in columns vary for the following reasons: (a) occurrence of non-response or (b) indecision of respondent.

The pattern of association between the three indices may be seen in the gamma scores in Figure 1. (In the calculation of the scores, the "don't know" and "other" responses have been omitted.) While all cells show relatively strong relationships, the highest is that between work status and the appraisal by the physician. This result may perhaps be explained by the empirical interrelationship between the two items. Returning to work on a full-time basis is often contingent on physician approval or certification to the patient that he is ready. In turn, the fact that patients are at work full-time provides an important fact for physicians to take into consideration when rendering a clinical judgment about capacity. What the patient thinks about his own progress is not as strongly related to either his work status or physician judgment.

Figure 1. Relationships between Primary One Year Status Variables at T_3

	Gamma scores[1]
Work status and physician rating of patient status	.80
Work status and patient view of progress	.44
Physician rating of patient status and patient view of progress	.42

Rehospitalizations and the Problems of Health Status

In initial tabulations it was apparent that patients who had been rehospitalized one or more times during the year differed on a number of variables from those who remained out of the hospital. While rehospitalization is not always a clear indicator of health level during the year, this item of information does indicate something of an unequivocal nature about the patient population. It designates that a particular sub-segment of men at some time during the period between T_2 and T_3 was considered sufficiently ill to require treatment in hospital as certified by the judgment of their physicians.

The event of readmission to hospitals serves as a means of differentiating two groups of patients in terms of health level: those who came to medical attention and who were sufficiently ill to require hospital treatment, and those who did not. (We are careful not to label these as sufficiently well as not to require hospital care during the year, since some may have had ailments that were severe enough but did not come to medical attention.)

In view of the importance of this rehospitalization variable, it will be employed in the analysis here as a control variable. Indications of the degree to which it distinguishes between patients at T_3 may be seen in the second and third columns of Table 1. In those columns are recorded the percentages based on cross-tabulations of the rehospitalization variables versus the primary status variables.

As expected, and as the two columns of Table 1 show, there is a high positive association between remaining out of hospital during the year and (a) physician appraisal of the patient at T_3 and (b) full-time employment status of the patient. The patient's appraisal of his own progress shows a weaker relationship to rehospitalization. The proportions of those with an optimistic appraisal did not differ markedly between those who were rehospitalized and those who were not. The chief difference emerges among those who were not doing as well as they had expected, with the rehospitalized showing a higher proportion in this category than the nonrehospitalized.

Primary Indices of T_3 Status and Antecedent Variables

Given this introduction, we can now turn to consideration of the relationship of antecedent variables to the primary indices of status at T_3. A series of cross-tabulations were carried out in which a broad range of selected items was examined. These were drawn from major dimensions of the social and psychological experiences of the patients, and they include social identity items also, as noted in Chapter 1. These areas are listed in Table 2, and include: marital status and family situation, work situation, formal religious participation, social participation, physical activity pattern, and patient optimism or morale. As already mentioned, variable selection was based upon the notion that these items formed an array of potential supports in the patient's "armory of resources."

The questions and responses which deal with each of these areas constitute only one way of assessing complex underlying phenomena. The data are presented here in line with our exploratory effort to ascertain the relative degree of association of each with the various primary status variables.

In Table 2, the associations are reported as gamma scores, with the significance level reported as derived from Chi-square tests. In the second and third columns for each primary index variable, the gamma scores are reported for the population, divided according to the "rehospitalized, nonrehospitalized" variable. Controlling by the hospitalization variable leads to some problems of analysis, insofar as the number in the rehospitalized group is relatively small. This presents a problem of insufficient numbers in cells, particularly in instances of skewed distributions of responses. In the table, therefore, it is indicated where numbers in cells did not justify reporting results.

Table 2. Association Between Primary Index Variables (Assessed at T_3) and Antecedent Variables. By Total Population and By Controls on Rehospitalization During Study Year. Gamma Scores.

Antecedent and Social Identity Variables	Physician Rating of Patient			Patients' Rating of Own Progress			Work Status		
	Total N	Rehos-pitalized	Not Rehos-pitalized	Total N	Rehos-pitalized	Not Rehos-pitalized	Total N	Rehos-pitalized	Not Rehos-pitalized
Age at T_2	--	x	--	--	x	--	--	--	--
Social Status:									
Occupation at T_2	.31 a	--	.26 b	--	--	--	.55 a	--	.62 a
Education at T_2	--	--	--	--	--	--	.48 a	--	.64 a
Total family income at T_2	.21 d	--	--	--	--	--	.29 a	--	.36 b
Marital Status, Family Situation:									
Marital status at T_1	--	--	--	--	--	--	.41 c	x	.58 b
Patient's marital happiness at T_2	--	x	x	--	x	--	--	x	--
Wife confidant at T_2	--	x	x	--	--	--	--	x	--
Index of marital disagreement at T_2	--	x	--	--	x	--	--	--	.48 c
Work History:									
Job satisfaction, pre-illness	--	--	--	--	--	--	--	--	--
Index of work stress, pre-illness	--	--	--	--	--	--	.29 b	--	.45 b
Social Participation:									
Index: Social participation at T_2	--	--	--	--	-.45 c	--	--	--	--
Number of clubs patient belongs to at T_2	--	--	--	--	--	--	--	--	.33 a

Antecedent and Social Identity Variables	Physician Rating of Patient			Patients' Rating of Own Progress			Work Status		
	Total N	Rehos-pitalized	Not Rehos-pitalized	Total N	Rehos-pitalized	Not Rehos-pitalized	Total N	Rehos-pitalized	Not Rehos-pitalized
Religious Participation:									
Pre-illness religious import	--	-.45 d	--	--	.29 c	--	--	--	--
Pre-illness church attendance	--	x	--	--	x	--	--	--	.41 a
Protestant	--	x	--	--	x	x	x	x	x
Catholic	x	x	x	--	x	--	.34 c	x	.51 a
Jewish	x	x	x	x	x	x	x	x	x
Physical Activities:									
Pre-illness frequency of walks	--	--	--	--	--	--	-.56 a	x	-.53 b
Pre-illness frequent lifting at work	-.40 a	--	-.30 d	--	--	--	-.58 a	x	-.55 b
Optimism:									
Patient view of progress at T_1	.33 b	--	--	--	--	--	.35 c	x	.41 c
Gains of myocardial infarction, at T_2	.35 a	--	.27 c	--	.22 d	--	.37 b	--	.32 d
Goal achievement at T_2	--	--	--	--	--	--	--	--	-.34 d
MD optimism/pessimism index at T_2	.50 a	--	.59 a	--	--	--	.47 a	--	.57 a

a,b,c,d: On Chi-square test of significance, $a = p < .01$, $b = p < .05$, $c = p < .10$, $d = p < .20$; -- = not significant on Chi-square test, or no meaningful relationship as indicated by gamma score; x = E less than 5 in more than 20% of cells. Gamma scores not used.

For a detailed listing of the values for all Antecedent and Primary Index variables employed in the analysis, refer to Appendix D.

Several major features may be observed in Table 2. The most striking finding, perhaps, is the general lack of association between each of the three primary status variables and the antecedent variables when data for the total population are examined. The chief exceptions may be seen in the relationship between social status and work status.

The patient's work status was previously reported upon in Chapter 3. In view of some repetition of data here, it is important to note that discussion of this variable in the earlier chapter centered on employment history as a separate sphere. In this present chapter the variable is used in the larger sense of indicating outcome in a major area of life. Hence, though some of the material may overlap earlier reports, the focus here is on the work variable as it relates to the patient's larger life picture.

Socioeconomic status is perhaps the most robust predictor of social behavior in the sociologists' armamentarium. It is no surprise, then, that employment status of heart patients was significantly associated with indicators of social status. Family income, educational level and occupational level were all positively associated with work status: the higher the levels of each of these variables, the higher the proportion of patients employed at T_3. Although these findings are not surprising, they have most important implications for the rehabilitation of heart patients. Similarly, a clear relationship was found between physician assessment and occupational level, and a weaker tendency toward association between total family income level and physician ratings. These indicate that the highest proportion of patients from the higher occupational levels and higher income groups were given Grade 1 ratings by the physicians.

Other antecedent variables related to primary status

variables consisted of (a) two linked to occupation, (b) two which reflected early favorable patient morale, and (c) marital status. Thus, consistent with the finding regarding the social status indicators, it appears that "lifting frequently" on the job before illness was negatively associated with employment and with a Grade 1 physician assessment at T_3. There was a positive association between reported pre-illness work stress and work status at T_3. The underlying variable, occupation, undoubtedly contributes to these relationships, since associations were found between occupation and (a) pre-illness work stress, (b) employment status at T_3, and (c) lifting frequently prior to the illness. Those patients who thought they were doing well earlier and who saw gains from their illness in a positive, constructive way were those who were employed and who received favorable physician ratings at T_3. A positive relationship was also found between employment at T_3 and marital status at T_1.

Those patients who rarely took walks prior to their heart attack were more likely to be employed at T_3. The meaning of this finding is not clear. No association between frequency of walking and occupational level or education was found in other analyses, hence we cannot make a simplistic assumption that the finding on outcome is somehow related to the underlying variable, "social status."

No antecedent variable examined was significantly related to the patient's own assessment of his progress at T_3 for the total population.

Thus, from these data on outcome for the total participating study population at T_3, it would appear that the social status indicators and those reflecting early morale or favorable assessment were linked to highest ratings on work status and physician judgments. The meanings of the social status indicators, since they also reflect distinctions between white-collar and blue-collar workers, is an issue which must be considered in interpretation. Review of this matter is pursued in a later section.

While socioeconomic factors are related to work status and some other aspects of the patient's rehabilitation experience, it is also important to note that there is no evidence in this study that these social variables are related in any significant way to subsequent morbidity. Let us consider hospitalization in the year after infarction—a major indicator of morbidity experience. Division of the study population into the rehospitalized and non-rehospitalized categories reduces the numbers in cells and reduces the possibilities for tests of association. For those items on which numbers were sufficiently large, however, some tentative observations can be made.

As Table 2 shows, for those men who were rehospitalized there were minimal associations between antecedent variables and T_3 status. While the matter deserves intensive follow-up, at the simplest level it would appear that those men who were sickest (as indicated by rehospitalization) were not distinctive in social status, morale, family situation, or any of the other antecedent variables. How well they did, as measured by the T_3 status variables, was not related to these antecedent items either. While we have no data directly bearing on the matter, given the nature of this illness, it seems appropriate to conjecture that the precise physiological course of the illness would deserve further refined study as a determinant of outcome status at T_3.

Those men who were not rehospitalized are, however, another matter. Since they constitute the majority segment of the study population, they deserve special scrutiny as the modal group. While their morbidity experience may not be associated with social variables, other significant aspects of rehabilitation are affected by antecedent variables. As we have reported, a series of associations were found with work status in particular. With the removal of the rehospitalized men from the group under examination, the associations with social status variables become stronger, as indicated by gamma scores. Further, a series of findings emerge which are provocative. For example, a stronger positive association was found between being employed at T_3 and being married at the time of the T_1 interview.

In the work area, those patients with most work stress prior to the infarction were employed one year later, again illustrating the influence of the underlying variable, occupation. The number of clubs with which one was involved was positively associated with employment, as were some indicators of morale. Patients who perceived early progress and viewed the illness as producing some gains were likely to be at work at one year. "Lifting frequently" was found to be negatively associated with being employed at T_3. This repeats the earlier findings on these variables in regard to the total population.

Reported pre-illness church attendance in the nonrehospitalized population was related in a positive direction to being employed at T_3. When religious groups were considered separately, this relationship was clear for Catholic patients, but not for those of Protestant and Jewish religious identities. In fact, the distribution on church attendance for Catholic patients serves also to account for the positive finding in the total population. These findings on pre-illness church attendance can be interpreted in many ways, and their meanings remain to be more fully explored.

Other items of note about this table as a whole concern lack of significant associations. Thus, in regard to the work status variable, it is important to note no significant relationship with such self-rated variables as marital happiness, job satisfaction, degree of informal social participation, and the importance of religion.

II. The Secondary Index Variables

STATUS AT ONE YEAR ACCORDING TO SECONDARY INDEX VARIABLES.   The secondary indices of status at T_3 serve as supplements to the primary status indices. In a sense, the secondary status variables are all drawn from the same dimension, that of the patient's perception of his physical and emotional status at one point in time. Since they are all based solely upon the patient's *perceptions* within each area, their focus differs from that of the primary indices, which are drawn from three separate sources.

Distributions of the patients' perceptions of each area are recorded for the total population in Table 3. They are divided also according to whether the patients were rehospitalized during the course of the year.

Looking first at distributions for the total study population at T_3, it is apparent that a case can be made both for optimism and for pessimism, depending upon the inclination of the observer. On the favorable side, 70 percent of the men reported that their lives had now returned to "normal," and only about one-fifth reported they were dissatisfied with their present way of life. Half saw their first heart attack as having produced some gains for them, and half reported that they were not ever depressed about their illness.

At the same time, on the negative side, over half the men reported four or more symptoms during the previous month, and half reported feelings of depression about their illness. Nearly a third maintained that their lives had not returned to what they considered "normal." Thus, within this set of responses no general pattern may be discerned, but rather a set of conditions subject to alternative interpretations according to the value system of the reader.

Table 3.   Secondary Index Variables: Status at T_3.
Total Population and by Rehospitalization.

Secondary Index Variable	Total Population	Rehospitalized	Not Rehospitalized
Index of Symptoms			
None	13.3	7.7	14.9 [a]
Low	31.1	18.5	34.7
High	55.6	73.8	50.4
Total Percent	100.0	100.0	100.0
Total N	293	65	228
Life Return to Normal			
Yes	70.0	52.3	75.1 [a]
No	30.0	47.7	24.9
Total Percent	100.0	100.0	100.0
Total N	290	65	225
Patient Depressed			
Yes	50.5	64.1	46.7 [b]
No	49.5	35.9	53.3
Total Percent	100.0	100.0	100.0
Total N	291	64	227
Maintenance of Pre-illness Activity Level			
Same and Increase	26.6	16.9	29.4 [c]
Less	73.4	83.1	70.6
Total Percent	100.0	100.0	100.0
Total N	293	65	228
Gains as a Result of Myocardial Infarction			
Yes	50.5	35.9	54.7 [a]
No	49.5	64.1	45.3
Total Percent	100.0	100.0	100.0
Total N	289	64	225
Satisfied With Life			
Very	22.8	25.4	22.1 [b]
Some	57.4	44.4	61.1
Not	19.8	30.2	16.8
Total Percent	100.0	100.0	100.0
Total N	289	63	226

Chi-square is reported for tests of significance of difference between
rehospitalized and not rehospitalized.

a = $p < .01$
b = $p < .05$
c = $p < .10$

When controls were introduced for rehospitalization in the patient population, some predictable results occur. There is a greater tendency for a negative picture to be presented by those who were ill seriously enough to require hospitalization. These men report in higher proportions more symptoms, depression, life dissatisfaction, lack of normalization of their lives and reduction in activity.

The responses of the rehospitalized and the nonrehospitalized differ significantly. Despite these differences, which are in accord with reasonable expectation, the responses may also be analyzed in terms of their meanings for individual patients. For example, though the rehospitalized patients reported symptoms in higher proportion, it is notable that the non-rehospitalized also indicated symptoms to a major degree. Half the non-rehospitalized were classified as high on the symptom index. In addition, nearly half of the non-rehospitalized patients reported experiencing depression in connection with their illness. One-quarter still felt that their life had not returned to normal.

These are examples drawn from the full set of secondary status indices which imply that the non-rehospitalized, in relatively substantial proportions, also had problems associated with their illness. Thus, although the absence of subsequent rehospitalization might indicate a more favorable health history for these men, their reports of symptoms, activity level, and morale apparently imply that they were still involved with the sequellae of the disease.

Secondary Index Variables: Associations with Antecedent and Social Identity Variables

Tables 4 and 5 present matrices of findings, including numerous categories which are blank, since no statistically significant findings emerged. The total matrices are shown in order to present both the positive and negative results of the computer analysis.

Though these sub-categories differ from each other in content, a limited pattern of association with particular antecedent variables emerges. One status variable, the index of symptoms, provides a patient assessment of an important aspect of his own illness, based on perceptions for the month before the interview. The relationship of work stress before the heart attack to subsequent symptoms is notable here. The appearance of symptoms is also linked to the amount of lifting done on the job before the heart attack. Although lifting is a characteristic of many blue collar occupations there was no significant relationship between symptoms and the various status level measures, including occupation. Another significant finding was that married patients reported fewer symptoms than the unmarried, and that patients with higher levels of marital disagreement reported more symptoms. Church attendance prior to the heart attack was negatively associated with the number of symptoms reported.

In general, it appears that early favorable interpretations about the illness and its implications are related to subsequent status at T_3. Those people who are satisfied with their life, for example, or who feel that life had returned to normal tended to be those who in the first interview in the hospital thought they were doing well or who reported at the time of T_2 that they saw gains from the illness. Patients who reported a low frequency of lifting at work before their illness (i.e., primarily white collar) were more likely to hold the views at one year that life had returned to normal, that gains had resulted from their illness, and that they were at least as active as they had been before their heart attack.

There was a tendency for some social identity vari-

Table 4. Association between Secondary Index Variables (T$_3$) and Antecedent Variables (T$_2$). By Total Population and Controls on Rehospitalization during Study Year. Gamma Scores.

Antecedent and Social Identity Variables	Index of Symptoms			Patient Depressed			Life Return to Normal		
	Total N	Rehos-pitalized	Not Rehos-pitalized	Total N	Rehos-pitalized	Not Rehos-pitalized	Total N	Rehos-pitalized	Not Rehos-pitalized
Age at T$_2$	--	--	--	--	--	--	--	--	--
Social Status:									
Occupation at T$_2$	--	--	--	--	--	--	--	--	--
Education at T$_2$	--	--	--	--	--	--	--	-.37 d	--
Total family income at T$_2$	--	x	--	--	--	--	--	--	--
Marital Status, Family Situation:									
Marital status at T$_1$	-.42 b	x	-.39 c	-.32 d	--	--	.36 c	--	.41 c
Patient's marital happiness at T$_2$	--	x	--	--	--	--	--	x	--
Wife confidant at T$_2$	--	x	--	--	x	--	--	x	--
Index of marital disagreement at T$_2$	.30 b	.48 c	.27 c	--	.57 b	--	--	--	--
Work History:									
Job satisfaction, pre-illness	--	--	--	-.21 d	--	-.28 b	--	--	--
Index of work stress, pre-illness	.25 b	--	.35 a	.23 b	-.29 d	.37 a	--	--	-.33 a
Social Participation:									
Index: Social participation at T$_2$	--	.51 c	--	--	--	--	--	--	--
Number of clubs patient belongs to at T$_2$	--	x	--	--	x	--	--	--	--

Antecedent and Social Identity Variables	Index of Symptoms			Patient Depressed			Life Return to Normal		
	Total N	Rehospitalized	Not Rehospitalized	Total N	Rehospitalized	Not Rehospitalized	Total N	Rehospitalized	Not Rehospitalized
Religious Participation:									
Pre-illness religious import	--	--	--	--	--	--	.20 d	.49 c	--
Pre-illness church attendance	-.25 b	x	-.28 b	-.21 c	--	-.25 c	--	--	--
Protestant	-.36 d	x	-.46 d	-.21 d	x	--	--	x	--
Catholic	-.31 d	x	-.36 d	-.35 b	x	-.43 b	--	x	--
Jewish	x	x	x	x	x	x	x	x	x
Physical Activities									
Pre-illness frequency of walks	--	x	--	--	--	--	--	--	--
Pre-illness frequent lifting at work	.415 a	x	.39 b	.44 a	x	.43 a	-.40 a	x	-.33 a
Optimism									
Patient view of progress at T1	-.23 d	x	-.25 d	--	--	--	.32 b	--	.32 d
Gains of myocardial infarction, at T2	--	--	--	--	--	--	--	--	--
Goal achievement at T2	--	x	--	--	--	--	.33 b	.65 a	--
ME optimism/pessimism at T2	--	--	-.20 b	-.21 d	--	--	.33 b	--	.38 b

a,b,c,d On Chi-square test of significance, a = p<.01, b = p<.05, c = p<.10, d = p<.20; -- = not significant on Chi-square test, o= no meaningful relationship as indicated by gamma score; x = E less than 5 in more than 20% of cells. Gamma scores not used.

For a detailed listing of the values for all Antecedent and Secondary Index variables employed in the analysis, refer to Appendix D.

Table 5. Association between Secondary Index Variables (T₃) and Antecedent Variables (T₂). By Total Population and Controls on Rehospitalization during Study Year. Gamma Scores.

Antecedent and Social Identity Variables	Maintenance of Pre-illness Activity Level			Gains of Myocardial Infarction			Satisfaction With Life		
	Total N	Rehos-pitalized	Not Rehos-pitalized	Total N	Rehos-pitalized	Not Rehos-pitalized	Total N	Rehos-pitalized	Not Rehos-pitalized
Age at T₂	--	x	--	--	--	--	--	--	--
Social Status:									
Occupation at T₂	.32 b	x	.25 d	.22 c	--	.20 d	--	--	--
Education at T₂	.22 c	x	--	.22 c	--	--	.20 d	x	--
Total family income at T₂	--	x	--	.27 b	--	.25 c	.30 b	.64 a	--
Marital Status, Family Situation:									
Marital status at T₁	--	x	--	--	--	--	.38 a	x	.37 b
Patient's marital happiness at T₂	--	x	--	--	x	--	--	x	--
Wife confidant at T₂	--	x	--	--	x	--	--	x	--
Index of marital disagreement at T₂	--	x	--	--	--	--	-.22 d	--	--
Work History:									
Job satisfaction, pre-illness	-.29 c	x	-.28 d	--	--	--	.35 a	.27 c	.37 a
Index work stress, pre-illness	--	x	--	--	--	--	--	--	--
Social Participation:									
Index: social participation at T₂	--	x	.24 b	--	--	--	--	--	--
Number of clubs patient belongs to at T₂	--	x	--	--	--	--	--	--	--

Antecedent and Social Identity Variables	Maintenance of Pre-illness Activity Level			Gains of Myocardial Infarction			Satisfaction With Life		
	Total N	Rehos-pitalized	Not Rehos-pitalized	Total N	Rehos-pitalized	Not Rehos-pitalized	Total N	Rehos-pitalized	Not Rehos-pitalized
Religious Participation:									
Pre-illness religious import	--	x	--	--	--	--	.20 d	--	.22 d
Pre-illness church attendance	--	x	--	--	--	--	--	x	--
Protestant	--	x	--	--	x	--	--	x	--
Catholic	--	x	--	--	x	--	--	x	--
Jewish	x	x	x	x	x	x	x	x	x
Physical Activities									
Pre-illness frequency of walks	--	x	--	--	--	--	--	--	--
Pre-illness frequent lifting at work	-.31 b	x	-.36 b	-.28 b	-.62 b	--	--	--	--
Optimism									
Patient view of progress at T_1	--	x	--	--	--	--	.33 b	x	--
Gains of myocardial infarction, at T_2	--	--	--	.52 a	--	.55 a	--	--	--
Goal achievement at T_2	--	x	--	--	--	--	--	--	--
MD optimism/pessimism index at T_2	.38 b	x	.31 c	--	--	--	--	--	--

a,b,c,d   On Chi-square test of significance, a = $p < .01$, b = $p < .05$, c = $p < .10$, d = $p < .20$ -- = not significant on Chi-square test, or no meaningful relationship as indicated by gamma score; x = E less than 5 in more than 20% of cells. Gamma scores not used.

For a detailed listing of the values for all Antecedent and Secondary Index variables employed in the analysis, refer to Appendix D.

ables to be linked to secondary index variables. Patients in lower occupational groups were more likely to report that they were less active at one year than before the heart attack, and that they were not satisfied with their way of life. Married patients were more likely to report that they were satisfied with life at T_3. Pre-illness job satisfaction was negatively associated with maintenance of pre-illness activity level and positively related to a satisfied view of life.

Depression at T_3: A Special Examination

Among the secondary index variables, depression deserves special consideration. The associations involving depression clearly should be examined in terms of the pre-morbid characteristics of the patient. Those patients who were depressed before the illness differ in their response at T_3 from those patients who reported little or no pre-illness depression. The appearance of depression in each at T_3 had differing kinds of meanings, one representing continuity, the other a new development.

As indicated earlier, in the present study it was not possible to obtain pre-illness personality assessments. In evaluating the T_3 response on depression, however, it is possible to employ retrospective patient self-assessments on the same item obtained at T_2.

To answer questions about the relationship between antecedent variables and depression, two types of controls were used: reports of previous depression and subsequent hospitalization. The term, "not previously depressed" refers to the response on the question at T_2, relating to the period before the occurrence of the first heart attack. No other implication is intended beyond this specific reference to this particular self-assessment item.

In the case of relatively small populations, use of

Table 6. Association of Depression at T_3 with Antecedent Variables,
Controlled by (1) Pre-Morbid Depression Item and (2) Rehos-
pitalization. Selection by Self-description of "Not at all"
on Easily Depressed during Period before the Heart Attack.
Only Statistically Significant Relationships Reported.
Gamma Scores.

Antecedent Variables	Depression at T_3, "No" on Depression Item Pre-illness	
	Not Rehospitalized (N=160)	Rehospitalized (N=45)
Frequent lifting at work	.67[a]	.77[c]
Work stress index	-.30[d]	.78[b]
Work satisfaction	-.38[c]	
Social activity level:		
Social participation	-.44[b]	
Religious attendance	-.33[c]	
Frequency of walks		.33[d]

a,b,c,d: On Chi-square test of significance, a = $p<.01$, b = $p<.05$,
c = $p<.10$, d = $p<.20$.

two simultaneous controls has the disadvantage of drastically reducing the numbers in cells. However, as Table 6
shows, it was possible to examine at least two groups of
persons not reporting depression at T_2 in regard to
associations of antecedent variables: (a) those rehospitalized and (b) those not rehospitalized. Those who
had reported themselves as easily depressed before the
heart attack were omitted because of small numbers in
cells. Hence, though we cannot characterize the entire
population, we can at least examine data on those men
who saw themselves as not easily depressed before the
current illness.

As the table indicates, among those men "not rehospitalized, not previously depressed," there were several
relationships between antecedent variables and level of

depression at T_3. The nature of the associations is such as to show that the men who reportedly were depressed at T_3 were those who indicated frequent lifting and low social participation. There is also a tendency for depression to be associated with both low job satisfaction and low religious attendance. These data are consistent with other findings in regard to the other secondary status variables.

Though numbers are small, some analysis of associations could be made for the rehospitalized group not reported as depressed at T_2. As the second column shows, among these men work stress and frequent lifting on the job were positively associated with depression at T_3.

ANTECEDENT VARIABLES: TWO SPECIAL CASES

Medical Prognosis at T_2 and Subsequent Recovery: The Sequellae of Optimism-Pessimism

In the listing of "antecedent" variables appearing in Tables 2, 4, and 5, there is one which is relatively distinctive from the remainder: the physician assessment of the patient at the time of the T_2 interview. While the other items are either drawn from patient response or are based on social identity traits, this item relies upon a series of professional judgments concerning the patient at one point in time. The physician assessment was used in Chapter 2 as a measure of optimism-pessimism, based on the clinical judgment of the physician rating the patient at the time, and it was a factor associated with medical outcome. In this exploratory study of patient status at one year after the heart attack, it seems useful to examine also the physician assessment at the T_2 period in relation to non-medical aspects of the life conditions of the patient. The review in Chapter 2 concerning the nature of the physician assessment and limitations on its interpretation applies here as well.

It is interesting to consider the associations between physician assessments and the primary and secondary status variables as shown in Tables 2, 4 and 5. The early optimism-pessimism rating is highly related to the physician assessment of the patients at T_3. Other variables related to physician optimism-pessimism ratings are work status of the patient at T_3 and assessment by the patient that his life has returned to normal. Related also to physician optimism-pessimism is the report by the patient on the level of his current physical activity, as compared with that before his illness. Here the maintenance of at least the same level of activity was related positively with early physician optimism. On the other hand, the early assessment by the physician was not statistically associated with the following variables: symptoms index, depression, patient assessment of his progress, perception of gains from the illness, or satisfaction with way of life. Thus, while the physician may be the best predictor of the patient's subsequent physical condition, he is not likely to anticipate other significant aspects of patient progress as far as this study population is concerned.

Personality Self-Rating Items and T_3 Status Variables

Another type of antecedent variable which may be examined here is the patient's self-perception regarding a series of personality traits. As will be recalled from the discussion in Chapter 8, this procedure was carried out at T_2 as well as at T_3. It was stipulated at T_2 that the patient rate himself as he perceived himself to be prior to the illness. These retrospective assessments can now be used in the exploration of possible associations between how the patient views himself in a series of personality dimensions and the primary and secondary status indices at T_3.

The larger concern is with the question of the influence of personality upon the recovery process. Is there variation between individuals of differing personality orientation in regard to the outcome of their disease or the level of their adjustment? While this question cannot be answered with our heart study materials, the data both from the personality self-assessment items and from the one-year status items permits at least a partial review.

The question may be thus rephrased in terms of more specific issues. We may ask whether components of self-image are linked to what becomes of the patient one year after the heart attack. It can thus be asked whether and to what degree particular self-image items are related to particular primary and secondary status variables at T_3.

Personality self-rating items from the T_2 interview were classified according to the three level system noted in Chapter 8. Code 1 was given to those patients who indicated that the item did not describe them at all. Code 2 indicates those patients describing themselves as having the trait "somewhat or "a little." Code 3 was used when patients described themselves as having the trait "very much" or "considerably." Cross-tabulations were then carried out with each of the primary and secondary variables, controlling as well on the rehospitalized nonrehospitalized variable.

Considering the data for the total population as shown in Table 6, it appears that two of the T_3 status variables are associated with a series of earlier personality self-ratings. There are clear associations between such personality characteristics indicating emotional ability, sensitivity, and drive in relation to the index of reported symptoms at the end of the year. Essentially these same

Table 7. Association of (a) Personality Self-Rating Items at T_2 Regarding Pre-illness Traits and (b) Primary and Secondary Index Variables at T_3. Gamma Scores. N=293*

Assessment Items: Rating at T_2 of Pre-illness Traits	Physician Rating of Patient	Patients' Rating of Own Progress	Work Status	Index of Symptoms	Depressed	Life Back to Normal	Gains of Myocardial Infarction	Satisfaction with Life	Activity Level
Sense of Humor	--	--	--	--	--	--	--	--	--
Sense of Duty	--	.20[c]	--	.23[a]	--	--	--	--	--
Stubborn	--	--	--	--	--	-.2_[d]	--	--	--
Angers Easily	--	--	.21[d]	.26[b]	--	--	--	--	--
Easily Hurt	--	--	.36[b]	.28[a]	--	--	--	--	--
Nervous	--	--	--	.32[a]	.40[a]	-.3_[b]	--	-.17[b]	--
Easygoing	--	--	--	-.32[a]	--	--	--	--	--
Moody	.22[b]	--	--	.32[a]	.29[b]	--	--	--	--
Jealous	--	--	--	--	.26[d]	--	--	--	--
Likes Responsibility	--	--	--	--	--	--	--	--	--
Dominating	--	--	--	.36[a]	--	--	.28[a]	--	--
Critical of Others	--	--	--	--	--	--	.22[c]	--	--
Easily Excited	.26[d]	--	.25[d]	--	--	--	--	--	--
Shy	--	--	--	--	--	--	--	--	--
Likes Organizations	--	--	--	--	--	--	--	--	--
Easily Depressed	--	--	.38[c]	.43[a]	.36[a]	-.2_[d]	--	--	--
Self-Centered	--	--	--	--	--	-.2_[d]	--	--	--
In a Hurry	--	--	--	.37[a]	.28[b]	-.2_[b]	--	--	--
Ambitious	--	--	--	--	--	--	--	--	--
Eats Rapidly	--	--	--	.17[b]	.25[b]	--	--	--	--
Hard Driving	--	--	.26[c]	.24[b]	--	--	.2_[c]	--	--

Assessment Items: Rating at T_2 of Pre-illness Traits	Physician Rating of Patient	Patients' Rating of Own Progress	Work Status	Index of Symptoms	Depressed	Life Back to Normal	Gains of Myocardial Infarction	Satisfaction with Life	Activity Level
Puts a Lot of Effort into Things	--	.23d	--	--	--	--	--	--	--

a,b,c,d: On Chi-square test of significance, a = p<.01, b = p<.05, c = p<.10, d = p<.20; -- = not significant.

* The "N" for each individual gamma score varies because "No Response," "Not Relevant," and "Don't Know" responses were omitted.

personality dimensions seem related to reported depression at T_3. For example, the following personality self-rating items were positively associated with both depression and the index of reported symptoms: "moody," "nervous," "being in a hurry" and "eating rapidly." In addition, data indicate that those who rated themselves as easily depressed earlier also rated themselves as depressed at the end of the year.

A different kind of picture is presented in the case of the variable, "life returned to normal." Here, as expected, there is a negative association with such earlier self-rating items as being "nervous," "easily depressed," or "in a hurry."

The meaning of these materials on associations deserves some brief note. In reporting associations we intend no inferences about causality. One interpretation of these materials is that the associations are the product of continuity in personality traits as revealed by two different types of measures. Thus, the more volatile, emotional persons, as seen by their own early self-assessments, may be once more describing themselves in terms of the underlying dimensions when reporting on their physical and emotional condition at T_3. The apparent statistical association may merely reflect the same underlying variables, rather than constituting a causal linkage between two separate phenomena.

Whatever the explanation, these particular status variables (or at least the personality self-ratings of 10 months earlier), may have some predictive value. In more practical terms, such empirical associations may aid in further identifying at an early stage those patients who are particularly likely to report physical symptoms and emotional difficulties one year after the initial hospital admission.

III. Primary and Secondary Variables: Interrelations as a Portrayal of Patient Status

We have tried to describe what happened to the patients in several life areas and to report on how antecedent factors may be related to differences between patients in their post-hospital experiences. We now turn to a third task: to examine the linkage between statuses or outcomes in the various life areas. If, for instance, a patient is "doing well" in one particular area, in what other areas is he also likely to be "doing well"? For example, if a man is employed on a full-time basis, what is the likelihood that he will be satisfied with life, or that he will have physical or emotional symptoms?

While such questions are complex and cannot be answered on an individual basis, they can provide some indications of the nature of interrelationships. In Table 8 a matrix of gamma scores is presented showing the inter-linkages between primary and secondary status variables. We have thus far viewed "status at T_3" in terms of some sub-components as measured by the status indicators. The materials in Table 8 show how these sub-components are related to one another.

On the whole, the gamma scores present a consistent picture. Thus, there is a positive relationship, for example, between being employed, having a view that life has returned to normal, having a favorable view of progress, and being satisfied with life at present. Depression, on the other hand, is negatively related to all these factors. Reported depression, however, was positively associated with the number of symptoms of illness reported in the previous month. In a sense, therefore, a particular rating on one variable serves also as a predictive indicator for other variables, and the gamma scores indicate the relative strength of association.

These data on the associations between status indi-

Table 8. Associations between Status Index Variables at T_3, One Year after First Hospital Admission. Chi-square Significance Levels and Gamma Scores. N=293*

Key Outcome Variables	1	2	3	4	5	6	7	8	9
1. Patient View of Progress	—								
2. Work Status	** .44	—							
3. M.D. View of Recovery	** .42	** .80	—						
4. Frequency of Symptoms	**-.33	**-.70	**-.49	—					
5. Patient Depressed	**-.53	**-.46	**-.38	** .66	—				
6. Life Return to Normal	** .67	** .69	** .65	**-.74	**-.81	—			
7. Maintenance of Pre-illness Activity Level	*** .29	** .60	** .63	**-.52	**-.34	** .63	—		
8. Gains of Myocardial Infarction	** .23	*** .25	** .36	N.S.	N.S.	*** .29	N.S.	—	
9. Satisfied with Life at Present	** .36	** .50	** .31	**-.27	**-.39	** .65	N.S.	***.26	—

* The "N" for each individual gamma score varies because "No Response," "Not Relevant," and "Don't Know" responses were omitted.

** p<.01

*** p<.05

N.S. = not significant

cators at T_3 are presented here in order to help round out the picture of patients as they are at one year after the heart attack. Since they are all deliberately drawn upon as indicators of status in the larger dimension of "patient condition," they may all be assumed to be inter-related by their very nature.

As we have seen, they are drawn from differing types of subjective and objective indicators, and they touch the physical and emotional dimensions of the patient's life. This portrayal through the matrix provides some rough measures of patient condition at a point in time. Altogether, they provide one kind of portrayal of the multidimensional nature of whatever one may call patient condition at one year: status, adjustment, adap-tation, life style and recovery level.

SUMMARY

In this chapter, our approach has been to regard the status of the patient at one year as a multi-dimensional phenomenon, comprised of a broad series of elements. We have presented a series of data concerning two thematic issues. One has been the question of the status or condition of the study population in areas of their lives at one year after the heart attack. The second has centered on the relationship of antecedent and social identity variables to the statuses of the men at one year. We have thus attempted to examine some of the factors which may be identified as predictors. To achieve these ends, we have used a series of variables as indices of status in the various spheres of the physical, emotional and social life of the patient. These indices have been drawn from objective sources, from the assessments of physicians, and from the patients themselves. An important feature of this chapter was the presentation of tabular material on both statistically significant findings of relations and on non-significant outcomes of computer analysis.

A central theme in the examination of the predictor variables has been a continuing interest in the role of social and psychological resources. Are there differences in outcome at one year, according to support received from such major resources as family, the work situation, religion, and friendship groups? While the nature of support cannot be measured directly, we have employed indices as part of this exploratory examination from which inferences can be made.

The following are some of our main findings:

1. Within the total study population which survived and which was followed for one year, the majority of men were employed full-time when re-interviewed (76 percent). According to the rating given by physicians, about half were ranked as having minimal impairment (57 percent) and a quarter (24.5 percent) required some modification of their activities because of moderate impairment. Thus, according to two major types of external criteria, our study population was a work-involved, relatively active group.

2. In regard to a number of other outcome measures, the subjective picture provided by the patients was rather more mixed. A substantial proportion of patients did as well as they had expected (46 percent) and an additional number (35 percent) reported their progress was better than they had expected. Moreover, substantial proportions expressed satisfaction with their way of life at present, felt life had returned to normal, interpreted their illness as having brought some gains for them, and reported themselves never depressed over the illness. This favorable picture has its "less happy" aspects, however. As the data have shown, substantial proportions also expressed negative views of their illness, referring to

high occurrence of symptoms, feelings of depression, and lessening of activity level. Thus, though generally well rated by physicians and though back at work, the subjective picture for the total population was not a uniformly optimistic one at one year.

3. A primary distinguishing variable associated with status at one year was further serious illness, as measured here by the occurrence of rehospitalization. On the whole, in regard to work, physician ratings, and the various subjective indices, those who went back into the hospital for either heart or non-heart-related illness reported more negative experiences than those not rehospitalized. Here, too, however, the picture is not simple. Many of those who were not rehospitalized reported difficulties in work adjustment and physical and emotional symptoms. At the same time, at the end of the year some of the rehospitalized did as well as those who remained out of hospital, as measured by the various indices we employed.

4. When antecedent variables and social identity variables were examined in relation to indices of status at one year, two principal patterns emerged, both related to hospitalization status. Among those men who were *rehospitalized* during the year, virtually no antecedent or social identity variables were found to be associated with their status at the end of the year. Such data suggest that in the occurrence of severe illness it is the fact of illness process itself which is of primary importance in determining status at one year; the phenomena underlying the antecedent variables and social identity items are of less importance.

Among those men who were *not rehospitalized* during the year, a number of antecedent variables were associated with status index variables, including those antecedent variables relating to social status, work relations, morale, relationships with wives, and physician optimism-pessimism.

In particular, it should be noted that the social status variables are related at two levels with primary and secondary status indices at T_3. These associations were direct in the case of several outcome variables, including physician rating, work status, maintenance of pre-illness activity level, and some aspects of patient morale. In other cases, social status may have functioned as an underlying variable, contributing to relationships between other antecedent variables and outcome variables. Examples of this phenomenon include: (1) the negative relationships found between frequent lifting prior to the heart attack and (a) patient employment at one year and (b) morale at T_3, and (2) the positive association between pre-illness work stress and T_3 work status. In our previous work, frequent lifting was seen as a characteristic of blue-collar workers, and reported pre-illness work stress was found to be reported in higher proportion by men in professional, executive, and administrative occupations.

In addition to the relationships already mentioned, some personality self-ratings which the patients made after discharge from hospital were also associated with their year-end condition, particularly in the areas of symptom level and depression. Not all these relationships were consistent for all outcome variables at T_3. Moreover, some antecedent variables, contrary to expectation, showed no association whatever with outcome. The consistent patterning overall may lend indications strong enough to warrant further testing, however. It suggests that, in the absence of further serious illness, the status or condition of these men one year after a life-threatening event may be related to the nature and use of social and psychological resources, as well as to the level of social integration of the men themselves.

An important additional feature of these data is that the findings for the non-rehospitalized men are also commonly reflected in the findings for the total population. The reason for this is that the non-rehospitalized group constituted a large proportion (over 75 percent) of the total population. Hence, when various statistical relationships are examined in regard to the total population, many of the findings are really due to the high representation of the non-rehospitalized in the total population.

5. Interrelations of the primary and secondary status indices at year-end showed a consistent pattern of association. Thus, those patients employed full-time also tended to receive higher ratings from their physicians and to show higher morale, as compared to those in a part-time or unemployed status. Those patients who were depressed also reported higher symptom levels, lower morale, less activity than before the illness, and a feeling that life had not yet returned to normal. These data show in their consistency some promise of predictability from one area of life to another.

In conclusion, let us note the larger trends. Approximately one year before the final interview for this research, in the areas of Greater Boston and Worcester, Massachusetts, a number of men were fully involved in their lives, and were without previous illness. When struck down and hospitalized for a first myocardial infarction, these men brought with them various resources and capacities of a physical, psychological and social nature. While most of these men were reemployed full-time at the end of a year, they presented a varied picture in areas of their lives other than the work situation. For those who remained well enough and were not rehospitalized, these varied resources and capacities appeared to play an important and complex role in how they were doing at one year.

This chapter has been concerned with but one segment of these sequellae of the illness and of the antecedent factors. In the next chapter we will review the evidence drawn from all the dimensions covered in this report. We will then move to an overview of their larger meanings and implications for patients, for those providing care, and for students of social process.

NOTES

1. Results of separate chi-square tests which were carried out for the above associations were as follows:

    Work status and physician rating of patient status—Chi-square = 115.07, df = 4, p < .001,

    Work status and patient view of progress—Chi-square = 32.29, df = 4, p < .001,

    Physician rating of patient status and patient view of progress—Chi-square = 25.41, df = 4, p < .001.

2. For a description of the personality self-rating items, refer to Note 4, Chapter 1.

Chapter 10

SUMMARY AND IMPLICATIONS

INTRODUCTION

In conducting our study of heart patients, we have been guided by a number of larger issues related to patient behavior and some practical aspects of medical care planning. In this final chapter we attempt to draw together some of the more significant findings and to review their implications for patient care and the sociological aspects of rehabilitation.

The materials are presented in three sections. In Part I we review the principal findings, particularly as these relate to outcome, life problems, and use of services and professionals.

Part II is concerned with some issues which emerge from these data in regard to the development of further research and in the planning of therapeutic programs. These include problems in conceptualization of the illness process, including those of definition, measurement, and the selection of relevant critical indices. We also focus upon such problems as the rational development of standards of care, definition of areas of responsibility, measurement of outcome, and other issues in planning for patient care.

Finally, Part III is concerned with some elements of the patient experience, particularly as these pertain to the care and rehabilitation of the individual heart patient. Here we consider some bases for patient adherence to the therapeutic regimen, barriers to communication, problems of differing role expectations for the patient, and complications which may arise as patients obtain care in the bureaucratic complex of hospitals and other health organizations. While the focus is primarily upon the individual patient and the barriers which may impede his recovery and rehabilitation, we also consider ways of handling these problems and situations more effectively.

The questions we have asked include: What happens to men who have been living normal lives when they experience a first life-threatening episode of major illness? What is the nature of their subsequent experience in major areas of their lives? What factors influence their lives after a limited period of time—in this case, one year?

In answering these questions, we have viewed man as a coping creature who possesses a set of resources and capacities which enable him to deal with life contingencies. The resources have been considered as an armory upon which men can draw, and we have considered them at several levels. These are: (a) the personal resources: the various physical and psychological mechanisms by which he responds to life crisis situations; (b) the social institutional supports, such as family, work, religion, social grouping; and (c) the organized institutions for care such as hospitals, agencies and other professionals who may serve as supports in an industrialized urban society.

This framework rests upon a view of illness as an event occurring within a complex social and cultural context, one in which the various systems in which a person is involved are interrelated. These systems present to the individual a broad range of potential resources upon which he can draw. At the same time, the individual exerts influences upon the systems. Thus, while a family may provide a support during illness, the sick individual, in turn, influences the form and activities of his family, affecting its capacity and willingness to provide support.

From this perspective, illness is viewed as only one type of life crisis event. It stands along with those many others which people may normally face in their lives, such as bereavement, loss of job and disappointment in love. Here our concern is with this life event as a stressor whose sequellae we may observe and record. The approach is optimistic, for it centers not on how the disease disables and kills, but upon the ways in which the heart patients deal with the disease and their new life situations.

The patients in our study come from a metropolitan area of the northeast United States. They live in an area notable for its concentration of medical facilities and educational institutions. It shares with other American metropolitan areas such traits as urban occupations, rapid communication, rapid transportation and a heterogeneous ethnic population. While our description and generalizations are specific only to the patients studied, these data and life experiences may provide a base with which other populations in similar stress situations and in other geographic areas may be compared.

Given this frame, we have focused upon various aspects of the illness crisis experience and on some larger issues of coping with life trauma. Our approach has been a descriptive one in order to document phenomena and their possible correlates, and our main purpose has been to provide empirical data on some issues for which little systematic information exists. The aim has been to generate hypotheses rather than to test them. Therefore, we have sometimes been liberal in our interpretations and descriptions, preferring to record as full a portrayal as possible.

The Study Population

To fulfill the aims of studying men in a crisis situation, we selected men who had experienced a first heart attack. None had experienced any previous major illness. Thus, this was for all a roughly equivalent experience: a first experience with a life-threatening illness. The age range 30 to 60 was chosen, since this presupposed a population heavily involved in life's activities. It excluded those who were retired or considering retirement, as well as those facing the problems of advanced age.

As indicated in the Methods section (see Appendix), the selection criteria specifying men previously free of major illness posed serious difficulties in obtaining a study population of sufficient size within a reasonable time period. The occurrence of first infarction is relatively uncommon in men under 60 who have not previously been diagnosed as having major symptoms of illness. Hence, it was necessary to develop an elaborate means of case-finding and screening. This was accomplished through the cooperation of 26 hospitals and through the participation of a staff of physicians as case finders. We were thereby able to gain the participation of a study population whose adjustments, problems, and prospects could be examined over time.

Because of the special nature of the criteria, however, these may not be construed as typical heart patients. Rather, they are an elite group in many respects: they survived the critical first days and left the hospital. As men without major previous illness, they were, on the whole, persons with relatively favorable medical prognosis. As men in the full activity of their lives, they had much to live for. Given their initial favorable situations, the problems and prospects that they faced and dealt with provide somber implications for the more typical and less fortunate general population of heart patients.

I. SOME FINDINGS IN REVIEW

Medical Fate in the Study Year

At the time of follow-up, a little more than 11 months after hospital discharge, about one-fourth of the patients had been seriously ill to the point of requiring one or more additional hospitalizations. This group includes a small number (16) who died. In addition, approximately 25 percent were described by their physicians as having developed additional significant disease processes. Within the remaining group, either no additional disease was reported, or there was insufficient information for various reasons, as explained in Chapter 2.

Was it possible to predict from early information which of the patients would require subsequent rehospitalization during the next 11 months? It was somewhat surprising to learn that the indices of social and psychological status in this study proved to have little apparent predictive value. Hypotheses abound concerning the etiology of heart disease, and we were interested in exploring some possible correlates of rehospitalization. Social status, occupation, education, age, stress at work, and some personality characteristics were examined in a general screening effort, but they did not prove to be effective predictors of rehospitalization during the study year.

A sole limited predictor appeared to be the clinical judgment of the physicians providing care. Their pessimistic appraisals proved to be most accurate: those for whom they forecast impairment turned out to have the most difficulty; over half died or were rehospitalized during the year. On the other hand, of those with the most "favorable" ratings, one-fifth died or were rehospitalized.

It should be emphasized that the period of risk was a relatively short one. Over the course of several years, for example, some of the variables examined might indeed be related to outcome. It should also be acknowledged that some of the predictions by physicians were perhaps less "predictive" than they were descriptions of a continuing disease process. That is, at the time of the questionnaire completed by physicians, those who were already exhibiting serious signs of illness might reasonably be expected to continue to manifest these, given the chronic nature of the disease.

In any event, since we found few significant correlates of severe illness, as indicated by rehospitalization, it was not necessary to control for more than illness level in our further analyses.

Outcome at One Year: Constellations of Statuses

The measurement of the patients' conditions at the end of the year was achieved through the conceptualization of a *series of statuses* such as work, marital status, classification by the physician, emotional condition and self-image. These statuses, when measured through various indices, provide a means of appraising the total life pattern and functioning of the heart patient that must be considered in looking at the nature of recovery. We thus go beyond such simple criteria as physiological status and subjective reports of symptoms, important as those may be.

What variables were related to the indices of statuses at one year? The selection of the antecedent variables, as the earlier sections of this book show, was guided by the conception of the armory of resources. We assumed that the family, the work setting, informal social groupings, the religious institution, and personality defense mechanisms could offer possible supports for patients.

We will not review in detail here the theoretical bases underlying selection of the areas. For purposes of exploration, we made a series of assumptions based on common theses about social integration. Some examples are: that marriage and family provide more support than unmarried, non-family status; that participation in the religious institution provides more support than non-participation; and that being a member of an informal social network is more supportive than being a social isolate. In addition, two other variables, age and social status, were examined. The "age" variable needs little explanation. Social status, a category comprised of education, occupation, and income level, was used in accordance with the thesis that position in the social structure is linked to life opportunities. The evidence concerning this most powerful variable is too well known to be reviewed here.

Instead of dealing with the population as a whole, it was most useful to divide the group into two sub-categories on the basis of illness experience. A simple though relatively crude differentiation was made by classifying patients as "rehospitalized" or "non-rehospitalized" during the year. In view of problems of diagnosis, variation in communications about symptoms, the denial phenomenon in illness, and other factors, it seemed that the simple empirical fact of being admitted to a hospital for treatment or dying of chronic heart disease seemed the most ready, reliable, and simple means of dividing patients.

An examination of the variables in relation to "outcome statuses" at one year yielded several principal findings. In the case of the rehospitalized population, a major finding was that none of the antecedent or social variables seemed related to statuses at one year. It appears that the fact of illness itself was the most powerful determinant of outcome.

In the case of the non-rehospitalized group, there were two principal positive findings. One was the relationship of social status to employment status and to the doctor's rating of the patients in terms of functional capacity. In brief, the blue collar workers tended to have the lower rating by physicians and they were unemployed or part-time workers in greater numbers. Further, the frequency of lifting at work (one indicator of blue collar status) was related to other kinds of problems, such as depression and various physical and emotional symptoms.

A second major finding was the relationship between the presence of symptoms at one year and such personality ratings as emotional volatility and depression before the illness. Thus, the nature of personality before the illness was linked to the pattern of physical and emotional symptoms at one year. Since personality ratings are not related significantly to social status, it would be incorrect to seek explanations in terms of emotionally volatile blue collar workers. Though the small numbers in the groups limit further statistical exploration, one may hypothesize that personality and occupational status make independent contributions to final outcomes of heart patients in this study population.

A third principal finding is of a negative nature:

other antecedent variables are not associated with the one year status variables. All these findings must be regarded with appropriate caution. The crude nature of the indices, the question of validity and reliability for both the antecedent and outcome variables, the working of statistical chance are only some of the factors which must be considered. Yet, we might also note that the positive findings are consistent with substantial bodies of evidence in both the social science and psychiatric literature. These demonstrate as well the general thesis that position in the social structure (i.e., occupation) and the pre-morbid personality help determine how well men do in handling illness, its sequellae, and the problems and experiences they have in connection with their illness.

Social Status, Illness, and Life Problems

One area of general interest in the study was the relationship between social status and the reporting of difficulties in matters of practical life management, such as work, finances, and family problems. After the occurrence of the first heart attack, it appears, the blue collar group, particularly the semi-skilled and unskilled, had the most serious changes to make in their working arrangements. As compared with white collar men, they were out of work longer, changed jobs in higher proportions and even had greater financial loss from being out of work. The insecurities of having to leave the old job and find another, coping with financial problems, and rearranging their lives in other ways thus fell upon this particular group. The data do not show that their difficulties were the product of their having more serious illness in the sense of more symptoms or higher rehospitalization rates. Rather, they are a reflection once again of differential life opportunities and resources of men at differing levels of the social strata. Heart patients are no more immune than other people to the persistent and pervasive influence of social status.

Differential Use of Resources

As noted earlier, for purposes of analysis and ordering of material, we conceived of three levels of resources: (a) the personal, including physiological and psychological resources; (b) social institutional, such as family, religion, informal social grouping, and (c) formal organizational resources, such as physicians, agencies and organizations of the community.

There was high contact between patients and physicians during the year, particularly for those seriously ill who required hospitalization. On the other hand, among the total population, only a relatively small percent made use of other types of personnel, institutions, and organizations. The reasons for not making use of these are complex and varied. This empirical finding must be considered, however, in making assessments of the relative role of institutional resources in illness.

Family as Support

The primary role of the family as a support and resource was manifest in our study. We also found that a type of surrogate family—friends and neighbors—also provided considerable assistance. Some variation in patterns of support by the differing sources were described earlier. On the whole, however, those who received help from one source were more likely to receive it from other sources. Thus, it may be that the more socially integrated the individuals, the more support they were likely to receive. Conceptually the support pattern may be seen as part of the larger dimension of social integration. Thus, in these data at least, the stereotype of isolated man in industrial society does not seem to be borne out. Instead, the family and "surrogate family" form resources which give aid through services furnished, through emotional support, and in some instances, through financial assistance. These were more important than the formal institutions and organizations of the society.

Religion as Support

Another possible source of support is that of the religious institution. We can assess only limited aspects of the role of religion in the lives of heart patients, but in terms of some measurable areas, several points emerge. As indicated by church attendance and reported valuation of religion, there appears to be no significant change among heart patients. This means that those for whom religion in the formal sense was important continued to maintain that viewpoint during the year. It also means that among those who attended church infrequently or who did not value religion, there was little change. While religion, therefore, may have provided support for a considerable segment of the patients, for men who did not value it before the illness, it was not a support to which they turned during time of stress.

Role of Medical Segment: The Physicians

Not unexpectedly, in this illness situation the medical profession was widely used. Patients saw physicians regularly and tended to keep a high proportion of appointments. There was no significant variation by social level in use of physicians. In general, patients appeared to have complied with the advice they received from their physicians regardless of their age or social status. Patients did not comply equally in all areas, however. For example, they showed a higher level of compliance in regard to taking medications as compared with changing diets. Patient compliance did not appear to be related to previous beliefs or attitudes. Instead, patients seemed to be powerfully affected by the critical life-threat of their illness.

Personality: Defense Mechanisms and Etiology

There has been considerable question about the role of personality of heart patients with respect to etiology and recovery. We were able in this study to examine some limited aspects of that complex construct, the "personality dimension". This was done through personality self-rating items as well as through examination of a series of other interview responses.

One feature of these data was the lack of significant difference between the personality items of the heart patients and that of a "normal" population, men in the Framingham heart study population.

The fact that the ratings themselves did not differ from those of the "normals" in the Framingham study does not support the hypothesis that heart patients have distinctive personality characteristics, however. Whether heart patients differ from other population segments in the United States has yet to be ascertained (Jenkins et al., 1971; Lind and Theorell, 1973; Zyzanski and Jenkins, 1970).

Some Overview Remarks

It must be remembered that the heart patients in this study were in a favored situation as compared with most other heart patients. They were essentially healthy adults with no prior experience with heart disease. Nevertheless, the illness experience of this population during the first year presents a more bleak picture than that which is popularly envisioned. As we have seen, approximately half of the patient group either died, was hospitalized or experienced additional serious physical symptoms. There were marked changes in the physical status of a considerable portion of those previously healthy men during the study year. One may anticipate that the picture would be worse for most other cohorts of heart patients.

This is not to deny that there are clear positive sides to the picture. As we have seen, 95 percent of the heart patients who left the hospital survived the first year, and an overwhelming proportion of them returned to work and began to assume their previous life roles. The findings on the physical problems of the heart patients in our study, however, strongly point up the need to anticipate the difficulties and to develop appropriate methods for meeting them.

II. CONTINGENCIES IN PLANNING

Issues of Definition of the Illness and Areas of Responsibility

As one of the most common diseases in the United States, heart disease requires great resources in terms of personnel and facilities for treatment and rehabilitation. The possibilities of developing preventive measures or "cures" do not as yet provide assurances that in the decades ahead the needs for these resources and facilities will be drastically reduced.

One problem in planning future services resides in the definition of the illness itself. In planning for personnel and facilities, is heart disease to be defined solely as a physiological process? If not, what are the boundaries of the illness? Do they include the total range of problems which relate to the illness and which may exacerabate it?

In this study we have traced the careers of 345 new heart patients for a period of one year. As we have seen, over the period of the year some patients had diverse problems, including new cardiac episodes, symptoms, emotional difficulties and employment problems. In the case of these patients, it is not always easy to isolate the purely "cardiac elements" from the total range of their life problems. Further, if some problems are not clear sequellae of the initial episode, they may be yet of another order: new sources of stress may become part of the illness picture. Further, even if the new sources of stress do not actually affect the physical illness, they are often seen by the patients themselves as relevant. One example is work stresses, which patients cited frequently as a cause of their illness. As long as specific stresses are seen as relevant by the patient, they would seem to be necessary to take into account in patient care.

A primary theme in medicine, from Hippocrates on, is the responsibility of the physician to treat the patient to the best of his ability and to serve the patient's best interests. Yet there are no uniform interpretations among physicians as to what may be the best interests of the patient. As the data on physician advice in Chapters 5 and 6 indicate, it is apparent that physicians vary in how they define the illness and what ramifications of the disease they consider to be appropriate for treatment. For example, some physicians may see family relations as an important part of the illness complex and one requiring attention. Other physicians may automatically exclude family matters from consideration. This means that in some cases family relations which in fact may be seriously troubling the patient, may be judged irrelevant to the illness.

In planning services for the treatment and rehabilitation of heart patients, we must make decisions regarding the degree and type of non-medical supports which must be provided, by whom, and within what systems of organization. We must also answer the crucial question: who should pay for the services?

A number of other related issues pertain to the role or responsibility of the physician. For example, how far should the physician and other health professionals go in the treatment of the cardiac patient in order to promote rehabilitation and reduce possibilities of another attack. The degree to which physicians should influence the quality of life of their patients also remains an unresolved and controversial point in medicine. According to one viewpoint, that of the noted cardiologist, Samuel Levine, it is useful for the physician to send heart patients back to work even at the risk of recurrence of the illness. Far better to die in full life activity, than to live as a cardiac cripple!

It is impossible at this point to reach complete agreement as to the proper role of the professional and the extent to which he should attempt to alter the overall life situation of his patient. Some operating guides or prescriptions will have to explicated, however, if we are to plan and develop effective health care programs. One canon which we might well heed is that the professional make his determinations in active consultation with the patient so that the latter's priorities may be respected as fully as possible. The image of the patient as a passive or mechanical recipient is no longer fashionable. It is also not consistent with our new conceptions of good health care.

MEASURES OF "OUTCOME":
SOME RESEARCH AND CLINICAL ISSUES

Research Problems

One of the problems which this study has addressed is that of developing appropriate measures of "recovery" or "adjustment". In this report we have attempted to sidestep the problems of defining those categories in favor of presenting empirical documentation of the "statuses" of patients in various areas of their lives. From the standpoint of pure research it is obvious that the measures used here provide only limited indications of a complex multidimensional phenomenon. In order to know where patients are in the recovery process we need to understand a number of key areas of their lives. Further, the relative importance of each of these variables needs to be assessed.

The task of measuring "outcome" is also complicated by the fact that some variables may not yet be recognized or identified. And some variables receive so much emphasis that, in some cases, other relevant dimensions tend to be overlooked. At the same time, other variables have been selected as major indicators on the basis of criteria which may reflect the value systems of investigators as much as they do objective utility. Thus, a variable such as employment status may be simplistically and routinely applied in studies as a key measure of outcome, while other areas such as emotional state, family life and social participation may be devalued or ignored.

To assume that employment is automatically indicative of favorable status in other areas of life is to have a simplistic view of the complexities and subtleties of the human experience. The fact that a patient is back at work, while superficially indicating that he is well enough to be employed, may mask a wide variety of phcnomena which are not necessarily positive. For some patients, returning to the same type of employment or to the same place of employment may mean a return to physically or emotionally stressful environments which may exacerbate his condition. Further, as reported earlier, a considerable proportion of patients believe that their work situations were important in triggering their illnesses. Hence, their return to work may mean their reentry into a situation of anxiety and concern—one which they may perceive as potentially lethal.

Finally, the phenomenon of denial, which is not clearly understood, may operate in the work situation. A proportion of patients, unwilling to view themselves as handicapped or as different from their fellow workers, may go beyond their normal capacities and undertake physical tasks and responsibilities which may literally lead to their deaths. This is not to say that for most heart patients work should be viewed apprehensively. But it seems clear that it is rather easy to overlook the negative physical and emotional aspects and to accept return to work as a valid measure of positive adjustment.

The Question of Use of Services

As we reported earlier, aside from the hospital and their physicians, the patients had little contact with other organizations and professionals during the course of their illness. One reason for this minimal usage was the lack of referrals by physicians. Yet it is also apparent that some of the patients might have benefited from help and guidance from various personnel and agencies. One-fourth of the patients were rehospitalized during the year, and another fourth were described by their physicians as developing additional significant disease processes. The problems of work and finances, particularly among blue collar workers, have been described, and the prevalence of depression in a large proportion of the patients has also been reported. It would seem, then, that a number of patients had problems that might appropriately have been handled by other agency or professional services. If some of these problems were handled by physicians, could not these clinicians have saved their own time by making referrals? It is likely, however, that some physicians did not believe the patients needed these other services. Or, that they were unaware of where these services could be provided. Whatever the reasons, it seems that more patients might have benefited from additional support and rehabilitative services than actually did, according to patient reports.

For their part, patients not yet accustomed to their new status as heart patients would probably not have adequate information about services available in the community. There is a common stereotype about the bold patient with *Reader's Digest* information who suggests alternative remedies and courses of action to his doctor. In reality, it seems inappropriate to expect patients to make their way through the agency maze in search of appropriate services. It would seem that more attention by physicians to the possibilities of referrals might have provided useful supports and direct assistance to many of the patients who needed additional help.

Early Prediction and Identification of Rehabilitation Needs

In planning services, administrators must allocate scarce resources and personnel to those clients who need them most. If those who need help can be identified early, this will permit more effective use of personnel and resources, as well as possibly serving to prevent some of the more serious complications which might otherwise occur.

For a number of heart patients in this study there were early signs that were predictive of subsequent difficulties at the end of the year. For example, those who reported themselves easily depressed before the illness were particularly likely to have emotional difficulties; those who were semi-skilled and unskilled were more likely to have work or financial problems.

The ready identification of these two groups as more susceptible to future problems can help in provid ing early care and support. The use of a simple personality self-assessment test may provide sufficient data to direct attention to those who are most likely to have the more obvious problems of depression and anxiety. The identification of the semi-skilled and unskilled can direct special attention to patients who are more likely to have adjustment difficulties and life problems.

It would appear that greater attention could be given to developing more sophisticated methods of screening for potential difficulty in rehabilitation. For example, the emerging problems of patients at various points in time following hospitalization can be mapped out and classified in terms of such categories as financial, employment, marital, mental health and physical health. Through appropriate screenings, steps could then be taken to forestall, alleviate, or even prevent the occurrence of such problems. This does not mean intruding upon an individual's life, nor does it mean providing a range of services in substitution for individual initiative and free choice. Rather, for those patients who are likely to have needs for particular services, these services can be effectively mustered, and at less ultimate economic and human cost.

In a community such as Greater Boston where there is a proliferation of agencies, organizations, and professionals, it means bringing the clients to service more directly, earlier, and with minimal flounderings and guesswork. In some communities where there are minimal available services for support and rehabilitation in heart disease, the problem would be one of developing or expanding services. It should be added, however, that there are limits to the services presently provided in most communities. To properly address the problems of heart patients, particularly from the working class group, may require new legislation on a state or federal level to deal with such issues as sickness insurance, job training and other social services and supports.

III. THE PATIENT EXPERIENCE: IMPLICATIONS FOR THE THERAPEUTIC RELATIONSHIP

Compliance Behavior: Limited Prospects for "Negotiation with Fate"

In assessing the experience of the patients in our study, we were impressed by the capacity for coping exhibited by patients. A general pattern among the heart patients (with some exceptions) was that of adaptation and change in the direction of health-preserving measures. While patient behavior was far from uniform, the picture is consistent with hypotheses concerning the conditions under which people will change their health-related behavior. In the face of a clear and serious threat to life, such as a heart attack, it seems possible to change the health and work habits of people.

These hypotheses may be specific and idiosyncratic to heart disease, however. In studies of other serious, life-threatening illnesses it has been shown that taking medicines, engaging in dietary restrictions or following other preventive action may be haphazard. The medical regimen may even be ignored by groups of patients. For example, observations of adolescent diabetics and patients with hypertension suggest that serious illness conditions, per se, do not automatically insure that appropriate health measures will be adhered to.

Why the differences in response to perceived serious illness and threat to life? Aside from some of the factors outlined by Rosenstock (Rosenstock, 1966) and his colleagues, we hypothesize that the threat in most other serious diseases is subject to delay and "negotiation with fate." The man with the bleeding ulcer, if he does not conform and has severe recurrence, may still manage to obtain medical care and have a reasonable chance for survival. In other words, if the acute blow does come (and it perhaps may be delayed indefinitely), there are still chances for a favorable outcome.

In the case of the heart attack patient, however, there may be little prospect for rescue. The patient knows, having experienced one episode, that there may be no chance to modify the situation. In the time of a heartbeat—or in a few moments—he may be dead. The continual anxieties which accompany the contemplation of this fate, linked as they may be to the physical symptoms, may lead patients with this particular disease to be more ready to adopt a preventive course. This hypothesis about the interplay of magnitude of threat, immediacy, and capacity for "negotiation with fate" can, of course, be empirically tested. It is only cited here as one possible explanation of the high level of apparent conforming behavior in this particular study population.

Since the study was carried out with patients reared in America, the data do not reflect whether these characteristics are shared by persons with other cultural traditions. Heart patients in other societies in which fatalism, passivity, or belief in reincarnation are strong cannot be assumed to display the same degree of activism in dealing with the crises of serious illness. Indeed, there is ample evidence in the cross-cultural literature and from public health studies that there is considerable variation in responses to acute illness (Polgar, 1972).

In our own study population there was considerable variation in patient conformity with medical advice. The clinical experience of physicians reveals a number of instances as well as hypotheses for the lack of conformity. One physician, for instance, reported difficulty in treating such members of the clergy as priests and nuns. As heart patients, he found, they were more resigned to their fate and less willing to bother with medical advice than were heart patients with secular backgrounds. It is apparent that with most patients, however, the physician plays an important role in influencing patients to follow specific health regimens. The pattern of appointment keeping, the favorable view of physicians, as well as reported conformity with his advice seem to support this view.

Problems of Patient Denial, Anxiety, and Communication with the Physician

Psychological factors also influence the condition and equilibrium of the patient. In our study we encountered frequent anxiety, denial, and depression among the heart patients. These feelings may often be concealed from everyone but the most intimate associates. Few who know heart patients are unfamiliar with the expression, "Only the wife knows." Commonly this phrase refers to her observations of the personal anguish and frustration which the husband feels. It refers to the private face which is generally hidden from all but the spouse.

One common but complex problem in the treatment

of heart patients is the matter of sexual activity. In the interviews with patients and the questionnaires from physicians some interesting discrepancies emerged. As noted earlier, relatively few patients reported in the interviews that their physicians had discussed matters pertaining to sexual relations with them. A distinctively higher proportion of physicians reported having discussed such matters. It is possible that the physicians could remember the discussions which their patients forgot. Yet, a considerable proportion of physicians reported that they did not discuss sexual matters with the patient. Thus, whether we take the patient's recollection or the doctors' reports, it appears that at least half the patients received no advice on this matter.

Appropriate sexual behavior constitutes one of the most sensitive and difficult problems which patients must handle. Sexual activity is more than a physical act. It involves a man's concept of himself as a masculine person, and it is thus tied in complex and profound ways with feelings of personal adequacy and worth as a human being. It is also a primary source of anxiety. While on the one hand, the patient may be driven to maintain adequate sexual performance, on the other he may live in fear of a coronary episode and possibly even death. Thus, the sexual performance itself may be feared by a patient as being potentially lethal. To put the anxieties another way: because of sex, he may die, and the woman who arouses him thus may play a role in his destruction. While such anxieties may fade as the patient goes through the various stages of recovery, they represent painful and recurrent problems in his adaptation to the illness.

How can patients discuss sexual matters easily with their physicians? For some the issue may be so painful, or threatening, or embarrassing that they are unable to bring it up. Patients of varying cultural backgrounds, social class levels, and degree of education differ in their willingness to share their feelings with their physician. The physicians themselves may also have their own inhibitions, which limit their ability to discuss these matters with their patients. Few physicians receive sufficient training about sexual behavior in medical school. It is generally left to them as individuals to exercise their "common sense" and clinical judgment on these matters.

Yet physicians, like other people, vary in values, knowledge, and sensitivity to the issues of sex. Those who have personal problems themselves in this area, or who feel uncomfortable discussing sex may leave the matter alone. If they do discuss it, the advice they give may be cursory or superficial. Or they may wait for the patient to take the initiative, assuming that if the issue is really of concern to the patient, he will bring it up.

There are other problems of communication between doctor and patient. On receiving advice on the medical regimen, for example, the patient may not hear the doctor correctly, or he may forget or reinterpret the message. In turn, the patient reporting to the physician on his physical and emotional symptoms or his problems in following the medical regimen may also communicate ineffectively.

There are also serious instances of denial on the part of patients. Denial may be at an unconscious level and may color responses, or the denial may be expressed as deliberate unwillingness to tell the physician the truth because of fear of the consequences. Our discussions with individual physicians and audiences of medical professionals reveal their substantial mistrust of the reported level of compliance by patients. On the other hand, as we have seen, physicians report giving particular advice which patients fail to confirm. Regardless of who is at fault, problems of communication between some doctors and patients merit greater attention.

The Role Set and Differing Perceptions of Distress in the Patient

Another problem area for patients during the year arose from differing perceptions of the sick role. A common situation is a lack of congruity among the persons who interact with the patient—in regard to the level and extent of his illness. In addition, of course, the heart patient also had his own image of himself in the sick role. Thus, while the patient may consider himself reasonably well, his wife may view him as a semi-invalid who is merely masking his symptoms, his fellow workers may view him as only partially recovered and as requiring special dispensations on the job, and his employer and insurance agent may suspect that he is well and using the illness to obtain special privileges.

The consequences of this phenomenon are common and potentially troublesome. What may be termed as malingering or as an "insurance benefit illness" may actually be a consequence of simple differential interpretation of how a man should behave in the sick role at a particular stage of his illness. Further, the wife who perceives her husband as "well", who pushes him toward full activity while he maintains he is not yet ready, may feel extremely guilty when her husband becomes acutely ill again.

While the wife may perceive her husband as well, his relatives may tend to perceive him as still being a sick man. Should he suffer setbacks or death, the resulting conflict, recriminations, and guilt may rack family relationships for years.

This area in the rehabilitation process may serve as an example of types of problems in which diagnosis, airing, and supports might usefully be given. Awareness on the part of the patient as to the problems his employer, wife, family, co-workers, and others may have in perceiving him accurately may provide a forewarning which can lessen his difficulties. Recognition of the situation and the use of a preventive approach may have long-term favorable consequences.

Outcome Measures: Therapy and Planning

We have emphasized the need for research to develop more adequate measures of the sequellae of an illness in order to clarify the total situation of the patient. The problems of inadequate identification and measurement of relevant variables for clinical as well as research purposes are equally pertinent. For example, it is important for service and rehabilitation agencies to evaluate the effects of their activities. One common criterion is the degree of success in helping clients or patients, although other measures involving "structure," "process," and "outcome" are of great importance. The less superficial the information concerning outcomes, the better the agency can plan. The better the criterion, the more it is possible to reduce useless efforts, cut budgets, and make changes in the use of personnel. One general problem at present, however, is that assessments of agency "success" are based on relatively rudimentary information.

Similarly, in the area of physician services, it may be especially useful to have clear criteria in regard to what is meant by recovery or by rehabilitation. At present, even for the same case, physicians may differ in their judgments. Further, the standards appear to vary even more notably when patients with differing social and psychological characteristics are involved. For example, in the treatment of heart disease, do the same concerns about the importance of work stresses obtain for the lawyer as they do for the semi-skilled laborer? Is depression in the lawyer or the worker viewed as an indicator of malaise which requires the active attention of the physician? While there may be many exceptions, some widely differing standards are being applied currently as to what constitutes reasonable "outcome" or "recovery".

Given the prevalence of heart disease, it is inevitable that many physicians see persons from widely disparate backgrounds, from differing social class, ethnic, and cultural origins, and with different types of work situations and personal problems. What kinds of outcomes can a clinician realistically hope to achieve with these different types of patients? The physician's expectations and behavior are determined only partially by the patient's problems and the physician's technical skills. To a large extent they are determined by the physician's values, ethics, and personal predilections.

In the medical world at present there is considerable controversy as to the goals which should be established for the heart patient. More specification of desirable indicators of "recovery" would provide a useful check list for the practitioner. This would help to ensure that clinicians give more uniform attention to different life areas of all patients. As programs for health care develop on a national basis, it may become even more desirable to make treatment goals more explicit.

Conclusions and Some General Policy Implications

We have tried to present a factual description of the experience of heart patients during the year following their heart attacks in order to fill a serious gap in our knowledge about the recovery period. Clearly, the problems and experiences they have go beyond questions of physical illness and involve such social and psychological dimensions as self image, emotional concerns, work status, relations with family members and level of social participation. Although as many as 95 percent of those who left the hospital survive the first year, approximately one-half of the patients in our study had some physical symptoms or difficulties in connection with the illness. This finding suggests the need to mobilize services to provide effective health services to heart patients.

We have also seen that the blue-collar workers had greater difficulty during the recovery period chiefly with regard to problems of work and finances. The need to provide additional supports to blue collar workers is indicated strongly by our findings. Our study also points up under-utilization of other social and health services by the heart patients and suggests that physicians should be better informed about the relevance and availability of such services.

Medical sociologists and other health investigators have demonstrated that health status is determined less by traditional patient care services which people receive than by the social conditions in which they live and the health practices they follow—in short, by their "style of life". There is little doubt that the things we eat, how much we smoke and drink, how well we adhere to regimens prescribed by doctors, and the way we live all play an important role in affecting our health. We are beginning to appreciate the importance of self-care and are rediscovering the role of effective health education in providing patients with the knowledge and the skills to take care of themselves. Effective health education, in the deepest sense, may become one of the most important services which physicians can provide to patients in general, and to heart patients in particular.

As a matter of health policy, then, we would urge that essential health education services be included within the rubric of our health insurance system. Today there is little incentive for a physician, particularly one who works on a fee-for-service basis, aside from his dedication and humane concern for the patient, to devote time to educate the patient, to answer his questions or to help him develop ways of changing his style of life. It is unrealistic to expect physicians to devote time and attention to this most important area when they receive no remuneration, and their extra efforts may go unrewarded.

Furthermore, if health education is to be incorporated as a crucial service for patients, the physician cannot do it alone. He will have to rely upon a range of other health personnel, such as nurses, counselors, social workers and various health paraprofessionals. One prototype of a program to change health behaviors is found in the Multiple Risk Factor Intervention Trial Centers (MRFIT), which attempt to prevent heart disease among high-risk patients, i.e., adult males who are overweight, have high cholesterol levels, hypertension, and who smoke. The program uses a wide range of methods to modify the behavior and style of life of these patients. Accordingly, counseling is sometimes provided, as well as various forms of group discussion or group therapy. The physician alone clearly does not have the skills to modify the health habits and lifestyles of these adult males. It is ironic that, to a large extent, physicians devote much of their time to counteracting the undesirable health practices which are inculcated by advertising and the communications media. If programs like MRFIT were expanded on a broader basis to encompass patients with heart disease, the physician would be able to rely on other health professionals and health personnel. The services of these health professionals and personnel should also be covered by health insurance, in view of the risk reduction they would provide.

It is important to add a clarifying note here. Some people may recoil from the idea of an aggressive physician or counselor dictating tastes and habits to patients, even if matters of physical health are involved. All of us would prefer to have individuals make their own choices, so long as their behavior is not harmful to others. But in our view, it would be the responsibility of a physician to make a serious and sustained effort to inform his patients: not merely to transmit information casually or mechanically, but to get his patient's attention, to reach him psychologically, to provide him with realistic alternatives and, when indicated, to help him implement his decision to change his health practices. Physicians and other personnel will have to relate to patients on an intensive face-to-face basis and to consider their cultural values and preferences in order to find the most appropriate ways of informing them and helping them to change their practices. If a patient elects to depart from the ideal prescribed by the health professional, the latter at least has fulfilled his responsibility.

It is clear from our description of the experiences of the heart patients in this volume that we are concerned not only with the crucial problems of morbidity and mortality, but with a broad concept of health which includes social components. We have seen that the recovery process of the heart patient involves not only matters of physical symptomatology, but also feelings of self esteem, adjustment on the job, relations with friends and family and participation in the broader social community. We do not view health as the mere absence of disease but as the ability of the individual to control his life and to perform crucial social roles as worker, parent, spouse and citizen. Our health delivery system should be assessed largely in terms of the degree to which it contributes to the ability of people to perform their social roles and to control their lives to the fullest possible extent. If a heart patient has the capacity to participate in the community and to work on a job providing he receives appropriate social supports and guidance, in our judgment we are failing this heart patient if he is compelled to live an inactive and unemployed existence. This implies the need to provide social services and supports such as counseling, homemaker services, transportation and vocational training. In addition, a range of health professionals is becoming available, including nurse practitioners, leaders of patient self-help groups, specialists in teaching self-directed, behavior-change skills, nutritionists, physical therapists, and others.

We have already made some headway in providing social services to patients. An increasing number of physicians recognize that the patient is a whole person who performs different social roles and is part of a social network which impinges upon his health status. Thus physicians and other health professionals have learned to rely upon social workers to ascertain whether the job setting to which a cardiac patient is returning may be too stressful for him, or whether there is need to redefine family goals and responsibilities so that the physical recovery of a cardiac patient is not obstructed. Clearly, social services can enhance therapeutic objectives.

Unfortunately, too frequently the role of the social worker in medical settings is narrowly defined, and his or her skills are not sought unless a patient is explicitly referred to social service by a physician. Furthermore, the various services provided by social workers tend not to be recognized or covered by insurance carriers. In view of the increasing "chronic" nature of illness and the growing need which patients will have for various social and support services, it is necessary to assure that these services are also encompassed within health insurance legislation.

We have stressed the need to provide new types of services to heart patients, including health education and social and support services. We can expect resistance to the provisions of these new services from a number of health professionals who regard themselves as specially trained people who use complex and sophisticated skills to manage illness and pathology. They do not think it is their professional responsibility to "interfere" with people's life situations or personal habits. Some will also argue that personal health habits are so embedded in people's history and culture that they are very difficult, if not impossible, to modify. Others will even contend that we have no right to tamper with people's way of life.

We believe, however, that the measures we are recommending are in accord with the changing views and expectations Americans have of the health system. We have become more aware of the pressing need to provide primary care on an ambulatory basis, particularly to those growing number of chronically ill patients for whom, at present, there is no "cure." We have also begun to appreciate the importance of social components in health and the need to provide social supports so that persons can perform their social roles to the fullest extent possible. The self-care movement in the health field, in turn, has emphasized the significant role of health education, and it has shown how health education may help the individual assume greater responsibility for his own health care.

Thus, it appears to us that in the future, humanistic values, concerns about the rising costs of health care, as well as our broadening conceptions of health will encourage health professionals to address themselves more intensively to the social components of health care. These values and concerns should be reflected in national health legislation, in the goals of health care organizations, and in the curricula of schools which provide training to health professionals and other health personnel.

Appendix A

METHODS

INTRODUCTION

This Appendix reviews methods of the study including: (1) the selection and screening of patients and (2) the nature of the research instruments employed. In addition, it describes characteristics of the patient population, case distributions at differing phases of the research, and other features of the design and methodology.

Collection of data was carried out through a three-stage interview program. These stages provide a useful reference point by which the case distribution and methods of the study can be described. Stage 1 interviews were those carried out with the patient in the hospital about 18 days after his admission for a primary myocardial infarction. Stage 2 interviews were conducted a month after the patient's discharge from the hospital. They were timed to catch the patient while he was still in the early transitional period of coping with his new role as cardiac patient. Stage 3 interviews were conducted at one year after the attack. This timing was set so that the level of performance of all patients would be comparable after a standardized period of adjustment to the illness. For the most part, the Stage 2 and Stage 3 interviews were carried out in the patient's home.

PREPARATION FOR PHASE I:
SELECTION OF THE STUDY POPULATION

For reasons outlined in Chapter 1, this was a study of men 30 to 60, previously free of major illness, who were participating actively in their lives and careers when struck down by a first myocardial infarction. These criteria were designed to produce a study population suitable for analysis who were coping with their first illness crisis. They were rather difficult to meet, however. As our experience revealed, it is relatively rare to find myocardial infarction without previous significant illness in men in the age group specified.

To facilitate selection of a study population, specific criteria were delineated for patients who had had symptoms indicative of or disease predisposing to myocardial infarction. (The full statement of criteria may be found in Appendix B.) A set of subsidiary criteria were listed to account for most major illness contingencies. It was decided, for example, that patients who had had a well-defined, discrete episode of disease in the past which had not required continuing medical attention were eligible for the study if this episode had occurred more than three years prior to the time of the infarction. The criteria were designed to ensure selection of a relatively homogeneous population from the medical standpoint, of patients whose condition was generally similar in terms of severity and degree of complications.

Sources of Patients

According to original plans, the research goal was a study population of 500 cases. As the project first developed it seemed desirable to obtain a population of this size in order to assure adequate numbers for multivariate statistical analysis and to enable the use of such variables as social class level and type of occupation as controls. Some attrition for reasons of death, mobility, and other factors was anticipated.

On the basis of discussions with medical consultants, it was initially anticipated that the desired quota could be met by obtaining patients from several of the larger hospitals in the area. When the study was originally designed, consultants and hospital officials indicated there would be no major difficulty in finding cases fitting the strict criteria. Hence, we made arrangements with two large institutions for the channeling and screening of potential cases. These institutions were the Massachusetts General Hospital and Boston City Hospital. While we anticipated that these institutions would provide a large number of cases within a reasonable time, we prepared also to enlist the cooperation of several other institutions in order to shorten the case intake period.

One of the surprising subsequent findings, as indicated elsewhere in this report, was that the incidence of myocardial infarction in men fitting our criteria is relatively low. Hence, it became necessary to obtain the cooperation of a large number of institutions in order that the case intake period not be unduly prolonged and in order that a study population of sufficient size be obtained. Because insufficient numbers fit criteria, it was necessary eventually to develop relationships with twenty-six hospitals of 250 or more beds in Greater Boston and Worcester, Mass. The arrangements were made through the cooperation of the administrators and medical staffs of these institutions. (A list of participating institutions appears in Reference 1.)

Medical Screening Procedures

Obtaining patients for the study population involved several tasks. In order to maintain an effective and medically sound means of screening cases, special arrangements were set up in each participating hospital. These arrangements were overseen and coordinated by the medical director of the project. In each of the participating institutions, a "contact physician" was appointed. This position was usually filled by a resident or a fellow, although in several hospitals it was necessary to employ a private practitioner from the hospital staff. The contact men were responsible directly to the medical director of the project.

The physician-contact men received a small stipend on a bi-weekly basis. This served both to reward them for duties performed and to maintain their motivation for regular scrutiny of hospital intake records.

The contact physician screened all new cardiac cases coming into the hospital. If a patient fitted criteria for the study, the contact physician completed a form which summarized essential details of the case, including the severity and nature of the patient's condition. In addition, the contact man obtained permission from the patient's physician in order that the patient might be asked to participate in the study. The form was then reviewed by the project medical director, and he made the decision in regard to acceptance of the case.

The contact men served in other ways as liaison between the project and the hospital: they minimized the areas of possible disruption of ward routine, and they had no problem gaining access to medical records.

Further, they were able to answer whatever questions might arise on the part of patients, private practitioners, or project interviewers.

Cooperation from practicing physicians affiliated with the hospitals connected with the Project was excellent. At least 98 percent of all doctors approached by the case-finding physicians permitted their patients to be asked to participate in the study. While this method of screening and finding cases proved effective for our purposes, at the same time, it was expensive in terms of money, administrative requirements and paperwork.

CASE DISTRIBUTIONS: AN ACCOUNTING

Case Population at Stage 1

REFERRALS FROM HOSPITALS AND CRITERIA. A total of 555 men were referred from the 26 participating hospitals by the contact physicians. Although criteria had been specified, the contact physicians tended to err on the side of referring all patients who might possibly be acceptable rather than making a decision to reject. Accordingly, thorough screening was carried out by the medical director for the project. The large majority of case rejections occurred on medical grounds. (See Table 1a for distributions.) The final group of patients who completed first interviews numbers 414.

INTAKE. Although it was originally anticipated that the total study population would consist of 500 men, it became apparent that this number would not be achieved within reasonable time. Hence, a cutoff date was set for intake. Case intake extended from July 1, 1965 through May 31, 1967, a period of 23 months. Since the interview program was designed to continue for a year beyond the first interview with the last patient selected, this meant the entire period of data gathering, through the last interview, was approximately three years (July 1, 1965 through May 31, 1968).

Table 1a:
COMPOSITION OF INITIAL STUDY POPULATION

Eligible:	First interviews completed	74.6	(414)
	Transferred to Case Study	1.8	(10)
	"Refusals," outright and indirect	5.8	(32)
Ineligible:	Medically	15.3	(85)
	Geographically	2.5	(15)
		100%	(556)

Table 1b:
PARTICIPATION AND CASE LOSS PATTERN AT SECOND INTERVIEW

Eligible:	Second interviews completed: "core" study group	83.3	(345)
	"Refusals," outright and indirect	4.4	(18)
Deceased, between first and second interviews		1.2	(5)
Ineligible:	Medically	9.2	(38)
	Geographically	.7	(3)
	Non-whites*	1.2	(5)
		100%	(414)

*Because of the small number of eligible non-whites available to participate, the decision was made, for statistical reasons, to exclude them from the "core" study population.

Table 1c:
PARTICIPATION AND CASE LOSS PATTERN OF "CORE" STUDY GROUP AT THIRD INTERVIEW

Eligible:	Third interviews completed	84.9	(293)
	"Refusals," outright and indirect	10.7	(37)
Deceased, between second and third interviews		3.8	(13)
Ineligible:	Medically	.3	(1)
	Geographically	.3	(1)
		100%	(345)

The Core Study Population: From Stage 1 to Stage 2

Data from the first interviews revealed that 32 of the 414 men had ailments not previously reported. Another three men became "geographically ineligible," moving to locations outside the study area. These 35 men were eliminated from the study, reducing the population size to 379. During the time between the first and second inteviews, three patients died and 18 men refused, directly or indirectly, to continue participating. These losses further reduced the number to 358 patients, all of whom completed the second interview. ("Indirect refusal" is a term characterizing those patients who through various means avoided being reinterviewed. Their evasiveness finally led us to drop them from the study group. This category also includes losses through staff decisions. The decision was made to excuse patients from participation in the few instances where further inquiry might lead to personal embarrassment or problems in family relationships. See Appendix C for categories of case losses.)

Thirteen of the 358 men were later found to be medically ineligible or inappropriate for inclusion, and they were accordingly omitted from the study population. This group included five men who were non-white. The criteria for the study population initially had included no stipulation concerning race, for it was hoped that sufficient numbers of whites and non-whites would be obtained to permit meaningful analysis. Since so few non-whites were found who fit the medical criteria, however, it was apparent that it would not be possible to make appropriate statistical comparisons and tests of significance. Hence, the decision was made to include only Caucasian men in the study.

With these reductions, the final core population at Stage 2 consisted of 345 men. This included those

Caucasian men who completed Stage 2 interviews and who fitted criteria for health history, age, geographic location, and survival (see Table 1b).

DISTRIBUTIONS IN THE "CORE" PATIENT POPULATION.   As has been mentioned, the study population was specially selected on the basis of criteria suited for the original purposes of examining the responses of men active in their careers who suffered a crisis of first serious illness. It was not designed to serve as a random sample of all heart patients. Rather, the emphasis was upon developing a relatively homogenous population in terms of the criteria. Through the screening efforts some of the effects of intervening variables were removed, including those involving variation by previous illness pattern, sex, advanced age, and racial origins.

Although this population is not a "sample" in the scientific sense, the question of possible bias in selection was a source of continuing concern to the investigators. Hence, several types of efforts were made to ascertain whether the project was receiving notification of all cases fitting the criteria. First, the medical director repeatedly interviewed physician-contact men. All maintained they were reporting every case fitting the criteria. Second, two of the medical directors served as contact men themselves for periods in participating hospitals. The number of cases they found was consistent with that reported by physician-contact men in each of the hospitals given this special scrutiny.

Third, a special project was set up in order to explore possibilities of under-reporting. A nurse was employed to review records of all coronary cases admitted to three of the participating hospitals for the year immediately preceding the inception of the study. These institutions were: Massachusetts General Hospital, Newton-Wellesley Hospital and the Boston Veterans'

Administration Hospital. Data from this special study were analyzed by the medical consultant. His appraisal indicated that the number of cases obtained from these three hospitals during the study was approximately that which might have been predicted on the basis of actual admissions during the preceding year.

The case-finding procedures resulted in a study population of men who, in a general sense, appeared to fit the major characteristics of the geographic area in which they resided. Some indications of distributions in terms of selected demographic variables may be seen in the condensed tabulations reporting on the core population of 345 patients at Stage 2. (See Table 1d.)

The Core Study Population: From Stage 2 to Stage 3

The study population at Stage 3 (one year after admission) includes 293 of the 345 "core" group (see Table 1c). This constitutes approximately 88 percent of those who were living and eligible at the time. Thirteen of the 345 men had died between the second and third interviews, two were deemed ineligible, and the other 37 men were lost through either outright or indirect refusals. Our experience suggests that some of the 37 patients refused because, once they were recovered and fully re-involved with their lives, they were unwilling to be reminded in another interview of their earlier illness experience.

STUDY OF CASE ATTRITION. In the instance of patients who died during the first year, details concerning cause and circumstances of death were obtained by the medical director through questionnaires sent to physicians of the deceased patients.

In order to ascertain whether or not the case attrition made a difference in the development of findings, a

Table 1d. Characteristics of Patient Population

Age

	Percent	N
30-39	9.8	34
40-49	36.0	124
50-59	54.1	187

Marital Status

	Percent	N
Married	88.7	306
Never Married	5.2	18
Divorced, Widowed, Separated	6.1	21

Education

	Percent	N
One Year of College or More	24.1	83
Four Years High School	32.2	111
Three Years High School or Less	43.8	151

Hollingshead Index of Social Position

Level	Percent	N
1, 2 (Highest)	15.7	54
3	18.3	63
4	44.0	152
5	22.0	76

Religion

	Percent	N
Protestant	21.4	74
Catholic	59.7	206
Jewish	14.5	50
Other	4.3	15

Ethnic Origins
(Based on matching of parents of patient)

	Percent	N
British-Old American	10.7	37
Irish	19.7	68
Italian	16.8	58
Jewish	14.2	49
Other and Mixed	38.6	133

special analysis was carried out. The case losses at Stages 2 and 3 were compared with the rest of the study population on a series of variables. These included age, marital status, religious affiliation, occupational and educational levels, social class, anticipated work status, and a measure of "denial" of the presence of the disease. No statistically significant differences were found between the participants and those who became case losses either through direct refusal, indirect refusal or death.

SPOUSE/RESPONDENT INTERVIEWS. STAGE 2 AND STAGE 3.

At the times of the Stage 2 and Stage 3 interviews with the patient, his wife was interviewed separately. If the patient was unmarried, widowed or divorced, as an alternative, these interviews were held with a close relative living in the home.

Of the Stage 2 core population of 345 men, there were 325 cases in which a suitable spouse or respondent was potentially available for interview in the household. At Stage 2, interviews were completed in 306 of these cases, including 289 with wives. Three potential respondents were ill (physically or mentally), the other 16 refused, directly or indirectly, to participate. Thus there was 94 percent participation by spouse/respondents at Stage 2.

At the time of the Stage 3 interview, 240 of the 306 spouse/respondents previously seen participated again; 42 of the non-responding 66 were not contacted for an interview because there had been no Stage 3 interview with the patient. (We interpreted refusals by patients as meaning that neither patient nor wife/respondent wanted to participate further, and we therefore removed both from the study.) Three spouse/respondents no longer lived under the same roof with the patient, four were ill and 17 refused participation, either indirectly or outright. Some additional increments occurred, however.

Six respondents who had previously been unavailable for interview completed the Stage 3 interview. Their number raised the spouse/respondent interview population to 246. This represents 92 percent participation by the spouse/respondents at Stage 3.

DATA COLLECTION AND PROCESSING

Data Collection

The collecting of data at each phase was carried out through use of a series of instruments. These were: (1) interview schedules administered to the patient and to a spouse/respondent; (2) questionnaires completed by physicians; and (3) supplementary materials obtained through intensive case interview methods.

INTERVIEWS WITH PATIENTS AND SPOUSE/RESPONDENTS. Interview schedules were framed to develop information at each of the three stages. The first interview, at Stage 1, was relatively brief. As has been noted, it took place with the patient in the hospital at approximately 18 days after his admission. Questions were designed to develop information concerning the patient's perception of his illness, his appraisal of his problems of adjustment and his future situation after discharge, and the nature of the plans he had made for changes or continuities in his job, family, and activity patterns when he returned home.

The second, or Stage 2, interview was conducted a month after the patient's discharge from the hospital. The third interview, at Stage 3, was set at one year after the attack. Both the second and third interviews took place in the homes of patients.

The schedules for the second and third interviews

were similar. They were designed to obtain information in regard to at least eight major areas, in addition to the usual social identification and background data. These dealt with (1) family structure and interpersonal relationships; (2) occupational history of the patient and the duties of his most recent job; (3) medical care costs and their impact on family financial resources; (4) attitudes and beliefs of the patient himself in regard to heart disease in general, and his expectations in regard to his own position and prospects in particular. Information was also obtained regarding (5) past, present and prospective use of physician services, hospitals, and agencies for support and care; (6) the patient's perceptions of instructions from his physician and his level of compliance with them; and (7) formal and informal memberships and associations. In addition, some indices to measure life stresses, particularly in the areas of work and the family, were used.

The interview schedules at all stages consisted of standardized questions and probes as well as various check lists, "fill-in" items and multiple-choice questions. The items were tested in 28 pre-test interviews, conducted during the winter and spring of 1965.

The questions in the spouse/respondent interviews were similar in some respects to the interview schedules used with the patient. They were designed to elicit material on aspects of the patient's situation which he might be either unable or unwilling to furnish. They also provided another perspective on his problems from the viewpoint of an involved observer. In addition, they included a number of questions to determine level of agreement between husband and wife in regard to issues of health, finance, family relationships, stress, use of community resources, and the presence of other problems.

INTERVIEWERS.   The interview program was carried out by a staff employed on a part-time basis. It consisted solely of social workers, with the stipulation that each have attained at least the master's degree in that field. Interviewing of the type required for this study requires personnel who are not only skilled at eliciting valid responses but who are also sensitive to the appearance of emotional stress and other potential disturbances in the respondent. Hence a uniform criterion was set, specifying experience and level of professional education appropriate to the high requirements in dealing with seriously ill persons.

Although all of the interviewers had extensive casework experience, they were given special instruction by Dr. Croog in survey research techniques of interviewing. As each patient was accepted into the study, his case was assigned to an interviewer. Initial contact was made in the hospital after clearance with the patient's physician, as has been indicated. In order to maintain continuity and ease of contact, the initial interviewer was generally responsible for all subsequent sessions with both the patient and his spouse/respondent over the course of the study year.

PHYSICIAN QUESTIONNAIRES   As indicated in Chapter 1, some of the major interest of the study centered around the doctor-patient relationship and, more specifically, doctor-patient communication and patient compliance with medical advice. Further, it seemed advisable to obtain clinical judgements on the patient's progress to serve as additional indices of his status at particular points in the illness. Thus, in addition to the interviews, data concerning the patients were also obtained from the physicians who provided care.

Physicians were asked to complete two questionnaires. The first was filled out at Stage 2, one month after the patient's discharge from the hospital. The second was completed at the third stage, one year after the occurrence of the first myocardial infarction. Items on the two questionnaires dealt with such matters as (a) the nature of the instructions given by the physician to the patient in regard to physical activity, work, recreation, diet, drug therapy, and other matters, and (b) the physician's appraisal of the patient's functional capacity and the prognosis for the first year. Each of these instruments required only a few minutes of physician time. The information derived permitted the development of such sub-studies as (1) an analysis of factors related to the patient's perception and comprehension of the instructions he received from the doctor, and (2) a comparison of level of patient performance at the third stage with evaluation and prognosis presented by the doctor at the second stage.

Cooperation from physicians was excellent. Approximately 90 percent completed the questionnaires at each stage.

CASE STUDY. A special case study was also undertaken. A small series of intensive case analyses of patients and their spouses was done in order to develop information permitting greater analysis in depth of the survey data. These materials were designed to supplement those developed through the survey-research segment of the project. More than 100 interviews were conducted in connection with this effort. These interviews were carried out by Mrs. Roberta K. Idelson, a member of the research staff; the materials are being reported on elsewhere.

Data Processing

CODING.   While the interviewing was still under way, several volumes of coding instructions were developed and the coding of data from all the instruments was begun. In order to help insure minimal error in these materials, a 100 percent recheck was done on all coding.

DATA STORAGE.   The product of the data collection phase was the development of a large body of information which was stored on 65 decks of IBM cards. A series of tapes was prepared for use on the IBM 70/94 and the IBM 360. Analysis was carried out through use of the Data-Text program and through the Statistical Package for the Social Sciences.

STAFF COORDINATION.   As the study developed, its size and complexity required considerable coordination. For example, there was a contact man in each of the 26 hospitals during the entire case intake period. The interviewing staff, at its highest point, included 25 social workers on a part-time basis. While interviewing was still in process, a staff of six women was employed part-time to begin the coding. At the same time, a series of research assistants, numbering six at one period, was participating in data processing and analysis. The project staff also included a secretary-bookkeeper and typists.

SUMMARY

In this Appendix we have described the research methods used in the study. We have reviewed the characteristics of the study population, sources of patients, medical screening procedures, data gathered and the methods used, distributions within the "core" patient population, means of processing the data, and case loss pattern over the study year.

NOTES

1. Participating hospitals included: Beth Israel, Boston City, Boston Veterans Administration, Brockton, Cambridge City, Carney, Faulkner, Framingham-Union, Lynn, Malden, Massachusetts General, Mt. Auburn, New England Baptist, New England Deaconess, New England Medical Center, Newton-Wellesley, Peter Bent Brigham, Quincy City, St. Elizabeth's, St. Vincent's (Worcester), United States Public Health Service, University, Waltham, West Roxbury Veterans Administration, Worcester City, and Worcester Memorial.
2. Some of the questions included in these instruments were initially developed by Walter Johnson in his study of heart patients. The authors are grateful to Walter Johnson for his guidance and permission to employ some of his instruments. In addition, the authors have drawn upon scales and indices developed by other research workers, and citations for sources are indicated throughout this book as appropriate.

Appendix B

MEDICAL CRITERIA FOR PATIENT ACCEPTANCE TO THE STUDY

LISTING OF SELECTION CRITERIA

Criteria for screening patients who had symptoms indicative of, or disease predisposing to, myocardial infarction were developed by the medical directors for the project. They are as follows:

Arteriosclerotic Heart Disease

Those with suspected but unconfirmed angina pectoris of any duration will be accepted into the study.

Patients with definite angina pectoris of one month's duration or less will be accepted into the study.

Patients with definite diagnosed angina pectoris of greater than one month's duration will be excluded from the study.

Patients with suspected but unconfirmed coronary insufficiency, congestive heart failure, or previous myocardial infarction will be excluded.

Other Heart Disease

No patient with heart disease other than arteriosclerotic disease diagnosed previously to myocardial infarction will be included in the study.

No patient with heart disease other than arteriosclerotic disease which is diagnosed at the time of the infarction will be included.

Diseases Predisposing to Arteriosclerotic Heart Disease

DIABETES. Patients with diabetes diagnosed at the time of the myocardial infarction will be accepted into the study.

Patients who had diagnosed diabetes at the time of the myocardial infarction and are being treated by diet, oral hypoglycemics and insulin will be excluded from the study.

HYPERTENSION. Patients with hyptertension first diagnosed at the time of the myocardial infarction will be included in the study.

Patients who have had diagnosed hypertension but have not received treatment for the disease will be included in the study.

All those patients who had had previously diagnosed hypertension which required therapy will be excluded from the study.

GOUT. Patients will be accepted if the diagnosis of gout was made at the time of the infarction but not if made previously.

HYPERCHOLESTEROLEMIA HYPERLIPEDEMIA. Patients will be accepted with these disorders if the diagnosis had previously not been confirmed or suspected at the time of the infarction.

HYPERTHYROIDISM. Patients will be accepted into the study if the diagnosis of primary hyperthyroidism is made at the time of the infarction.

Patients with secondary hyperthyroidism will be excluded from the study.

ACCEPTANCE OF PATIENTS WITH "NON-COMPLICATED" CLINICAL COURSE.   Only those patients whose clinical course during first hospitalization was "without complications" will be accepted for the interview program.

Appendix C

CATEGORIES OF CASES "LOST" TO THE PROJECT

1. Ineligible: *On medical grounds.* Does not fulfill medical criteria. Includes both mental and physical illness. Course of cardiac illness in the hospital was other than "noncomplicated."

   On geographic grounds. Comes from out of state or moves to distant location.

2. Deceased

3. Refusal: *Outright.* Overt rejection of continued participation by patient (or spouse/respondent).

   Indirect. A residual category indicating possible oblique rejection of continued participation. For example, interview evaded, patient cannot be traced, opposition to patient's participation by wife directly or patient claims wife is reluctant to have him participate, evidence further inquiry might lead to personal embarrassment for the patient, etc.

4. Staff Decision on Eligibility: So few non-whites in the study after exclusions on basis of other criteria that, for statistical reasons, decision was made to exclude eligible Blacks (N = 5).

Appendix D

ANTECEDENT, PRIMARY AND SECONDARY INDEX VARIABLE VALUES FOR CHAPTER 9, TABLES 2, 4 AND 5

I. Antecedent and Social Identity Variables

a. Age — 1 = Old (50-60); 2 = Middle (40-49); 3 = Young (30-39)

b. Occupation — 1 = Executives and Professionals; 2 = Administrative and Clerical Personnel; 3 = Skilled Laborers; 4 = Semi-skilled and Unskilled Laborers

c. Education — 1 = 1 Year of College or More; 2 = High School Graduate; 3 = 3 Years of High School or Less

d. Total Family Income — 1 = $15,000 or Above; 2 = $10,000-$14,999; 3 = $7,500-$9,999; 4 = $7,499 or Less

e. Marital Status — 1 = Married; 2 = Not Married

f. Patient Marital Happiness — 1 = Happy; 2 = Average; 3 = Unhappy

g. Wife Confidant: Number of Things Can Discuss with Wife — 1 = Anything; 2 = Most; 3 = Some; 4 = None

h. Index of Marital Disagreement — 1 = High; 2 = Medium; 3 = Low

i. Pre-illness Job   1 = Very Satisfied; 2 = Satisfied; 3 = Not
    Satisfaction   Satisfied

j. Index of Pre-   1 = High; 2 = Low; 3 = None
    illness Work
    Stress

k. Index of Social   1 = High; 2 = Low
    Participation

l. Number of   1 = Three or More; 2 = Two; 3 = One;
    Clubs   4 = None

m. Pre-illness   1 = Important; 2 = Not Important
    Importance of
    Religion

n. Pre-illness   1 = High (More Than Twice a Month);
    Church   2 = Low (Once a Month or Less);
    Attendance   3 = Never

o. Pre-illness   1 = Frequently; 2 = Sometimes; 3 = Rarely
    Frequency of   or Never
    Walks

p. Pre-illness   1 = Frequently; 2 = Sometimes; 3 = Never
    Frequency of
    Lifting At
    Work

q. Patient View   1 = Better Than Expected; 2 = As Well As
    of Progress   Expected; 3 = Not As Well As Expected
    At T 1

r. Gains of MI   1 = Yes; 2 = No

s. Goal   1 = Beyond Ambitions; 2 = Close to Ambi-
    Achievement   tions; 3 = Behind Ambitions

t. M.D. Optimism/
    Pessimism Index 1 = Full Activity; 2 = Significant Modifica-
                    tions 3 = Definite Limitations

II. Primary Index Variables
    a. Physician Rating 1 = Full; 2 = Some; 3 = Limited
    b. Patient's Rating 1 = Better Than Expected; 2 = As Well As
        of Own   Expected; 3 = Not As Well As Expected
        Progress
    c. Work Status   1 = Employed; 2 = Unemployed

III. Secondary Index Variables
    a. Index of
        Symptoms   1 = High; 2 = Low
    b. Patient Depressed 1 = Yes; 2 = No
    c. Life Returned to 1 = Yes; 2 = No
        Normal
    d. Maintenance of
        Pre-illness   1 = Same or More Than Pre-illness
        Activity Level   2 = Less Than Pre-illness
    e. Gains of MI   1 = Yes; 2 = No
    f. Satisfaction With 1 = Very Satisfied; 2 = Some;
        Life   3 = Not Satisfied

BIBLIOGRAPHY

N. Adams, *Kinship in an Urban Setting* (Chicago: Markham Publishing Company, 1968).

N. Adams, "Structural Factors Affecting Parental Aid to Married Children," *Journal of Marriage and the Family,* 26 (1964), pp. 327-331.

C. Aguilera and J. M. Messick, *Crisis Intervention—Theory and Methodology* (St. Louis: C.V. Mosby Co., 1974).

J. Aldous, "Intergenerational Visiting Patterns: Variation in Boundary Maintenance as an Explanation," *Family Process,* 6 (1967), pp. 235-251.

A. Antonovsky, "Social Class and Illness: A Reconsideration," *Sociological Inquiry,* 37 (1967), pp. 311-322.

A. Antonovsky, "Social Class and Major Cardiovascular Diseases," *Journal of Chronic Diseases,* 21 (May 1968), pp. 65-106.

American Heart Association. Heart Facts 1975 (New York: American Heart Association, 1974).

M. Axelrod, "Urban Structure and Social Participation," *American Sociological Review,* 21 (1956), pp. 13-18.

O.W. Beard, H.R. Hipp, M. Robins, J.S. Taylor, R.V. Ebert and L.G. Beran, "Initial Myocardial Infarction Among 503 Veterans: 5-Year Survival," *American Journal of Medicine,* 28 (1960), pp. 871-883.

M.H. Becker, R.H. Drachman and J.P. Kirscht, "A New Approach to Explaining Sick-Role Behavior in Low-Income Populations," *American Journal of Public Health,* 64 (1974), pp. 205-216.

M.H. Becker, R. Drachman and J.P. Kirscht, "Predicting Mothers' Compliance With Pediatric Medical Regimens," *Journal of Pediatrics,* 81 (1972), pp. 843-854.

M.H. Becker and L.A. Maiman, "Sociobehavioral Determinants of Compliance With Health and Medical Care Recommendations," *Medical Care,* 13 (1975), pp. 10-24.

C. Bengtsson, "Ischemic Heart Disease in Women," *Acta Medica Scandinavica Supplementum,* 549 (1973), p. 28.

G. Biorck, "The Return to Work of Patients with Myocardial Infarction," *Journal of Chronic Diseases,* 17 (1964), pp. 653-657.

S.W. Bloom and R.N. Wilson, "Patient-Practitioner Relationships," in Howard E. Freeman, S. Levine and L.G. Reeder (eds.), *Handbook of Medical Sociology* (Englewood Cliffs, New Jersey: Prentice-Hall, 1972).

Philip Booth, *Social Security in America* (Ann Arbor, Michigan: Institute of Labor and Industrial Relations, 1973).

R.A Bruce, "The Benefits of Physical Training for Patients With Coronary Heart Disease," in Ingelfinger, Ebert, Finland and Relman (eds.), *Controversy in Internal Medicine II* (Philadelphia: W.B. Saunders, 1974).

J.G. Bruhn, B. Chandler, T.N. Lynn and S. Wolf, "Social Characteristics of Patients with Coronary Heart Disease," *American Journal of the Medical Sciences,* 251 (June 1966), pp. 629-637.

J.G. Bruhn, S. Wolf and B.U. Philips, "A Psychosocial Study of Surviving Male Coronary Patients and Controls Followed Over Nine Years," *Journal of Psychosomatic Research,* 15 (1971), pp. 305-313.

E.W. Burgess and P. Wallin, *Engagement and Marriage* (Chicago: J.B. Lippincott Co., 1953), pp. 470-506.

A. Burt, D. Illingworth, T. Shaw, P. Thornley, P. White and R. Turner, "Stopping Smoking After Myocardial Infarction," *Lancet,* 1 (1974), pp. 304-306.

L.D. Cady, M.M. Gertler, L.G. Gottsch and M.A. Woodbury, "The Factor Structure of Variables Concerned with Coronary Artery Disease," *Behavioral Science,* 6 (1961), pp. 37-41.

B. Caffrey, "Interpersonal and Psychological Characteristics in Cardiovascular Disease: A Review of Empirical Findings," *Milbank Memorial Fund Quarterly,* 40 (1967), pp. 119-140.

B. Caffrey, "A Multivariate Analysis of Socio-Psychological Factors in

Monks With Myocardial Infarctions," *American Journal of Public Health*, 60 (1970), pp. 452-458.

B. Caffrey, "Reliability and Validity of Personality and Behavioral Measures in a Study of Coronary Heart Disease," *Journal of Chronic Diseases*, 21 (1961), pp. 191-204.

Robert D. Caplan, Sidney Cobb, John R.P. French, Jr., R. Van Harrison, and S.R. Pinneau, Jr., *Job Demands and Worker Health: Main Effects and Occupational Differences* (Washington, D.C.: U.S. Department of Health, Education, and Welfare, 1975).

R. Cattell, *Factor Analysis* (New York: Harper and Row, 1952).

R.S. Cavan, "Subcultural Variations and Mobility," in Harold T. Christensen (ed.), *Handbook of Marriage and the Family* (Chicago: Rand-McNally, 1964), pp. 535-584.

J.M. Chapman, L.G. Reeder, F.J. Massey, Jr., E.R. Borun, B. Picken, G.G. Browning, A.H. Coulson and D.H. Zimmerman, "Relationships of Stress, Tranquilizers, and Serum Cholesterol Levels in a Sample Population Under Study for Coronary Heart Disease," *American Journal of Epidemiology*, 83 (May 1966), pp. 537-547.

E. Chen and S. Cobb, "Family Structure in Relation to Health and Disease," *Journal of Chronic Diseases*, 12 (1960), pp. 544-567.

S.E. Cleveland and D.L. Johnson, "Personality Patterns in Young Males With Coronary Disease," *Psychosomatic Medicine*, 24 (1962), pp. 600-610.

P. Converse, "Attitudes and Non-Attitudes: Continuation of a Dialogue," Paper presented at the 17th International Congress of Psychology (Washington, D.C., 1963).

E.P. Copp, "A Controlled Trial of Rehabilitation," *Annals of Physical Medicine*, 8 (1965-1966), pp. 151-167.

E.P. Copp, "A Further Controlled Trial of Rehabilitation," *Annals of Physical Medicine*, 8 (1965-1966), pp. 220-223.

R.B. Crain and M.E. Missal, "The Industrial Employee With Myocardial Infarction and His Ability to Return to Work: Follow-up Report," *New York Journal of Medicine*, 56 (1956), pp. 2238-2244.

Criteria Committee of the New York Heart Association. Diseases of the Heart and Blood Vessels: Nomenclature and Criteria for Diagnosis (Boston: Little, Brown, and Co., 6th Edition, 1964), pp. 112-114.

S.H. Croog, "The Family as a Source of Stress," in S. Levine and N.A. Scotch (eds.), *Social Stress* (Chicago: Aldine Press, 1970), pp. 20-57.

S.H. Croog, "Problems of Barriers in the Rehabilitation of Heart Patients: Social and Psychological Aspects," *Cardiac Rehabilitation,* 6 (1975), pp. 27-30.

S.H. Croog, "Social Aspects of Cardiac Rehabilitation: A Selective Review," in N. Wenger and H. Hellerstein (eds.), *Rehabilitation of the Patient After Myocardial Infarction* (New York: John Wiley & Sons, in press).

S.H. Croog and E. Fitzgerald, "Subjective Stress and Serious Illness of a Spouse: Wives of Heart Patients," *Journal of Health and Social Behavior,* 19 (1978).

S.H. Croog, M. Koslowsky and S. Levine, "Personality Self-Descriptions of Male Heart Patients and Their Wives: Issues of Congruence and 'Coronary Personality'," *Perceptual and Motor Skills,* 43 (1976), pp. 927–937.

S.H. Croog and S. Levine, "Religion, Secularism and Personal Crisis: A Report on Heart Patients," *Social Science and Medicine,* 6 (1972), pp. 17-36.

S.H. Croog and S. Levine, "Social Status and Subjective Perceptions of 250 Men After Myocardial Infarction," *Public Health Reports,* 84 (1969), pp. 989-997.

S.H. Croog, S. Levine and Z. Lurie, "The Heart Patient and the Recovery Process: A Review of Directions of Research on Social and Psychological Factors," *Social Science and Medicine,* 2 (1968), pp. 111-164.

S.H. Croog, A. Lipson and S. Levine, "Help Patterns in Severe Illness: The Role of Kin Network and Non-Family Resources," *Journal of Marriage and the Family,* 34 (February 1972), pp. 32-41.

S.H. Croog and N.P. Richards, "Health Beliefs and Smoking Patterns in Heart Patients and Their Wives: A Longitudinal Study," *American Journal of Public Health,* 67 (1977).

S.H. Croog, D.S. Shapiro and S. Levine, "Denial Among Male Heart Patients," *Psychosomatic Medicine,* 33 (1971), pp. 385-397.

F. Davis, *Passage Through Crisis: Polio Victims and Their Families* (Indianapolis: Bobbs-Merrill, 1954).

M.S. Davis, "Physiologic, Psychological and Demographic Factors in Patient Compliance with Doctors' Orders," *Medical Care,* 6 (1968), pp. 115-122.

M.S. Davis, "Predicting Non-Compliant Behavior," *Journal of Health and Social Behavior,* 8 (1967), pp. 265-271.

M.S. Davis, "Variations in Patients' Compliance with Doctors' Advice: An Empirical Analysis of Patterns of Communication," *American Journal of Public Health,* 58 (1968), pp. 274-287.

M.S. Davis and R. L. Eichhorn, "Compliance with Medical Regimens:

A Panel Study," *Journal of Health and Human Behavior*, 4 (1963), pp. 240-249.

T.R. Dawber, F.E. Moore and G.V. Mann, "Coronary Heart Disease in the Framingham Study," *American Journal of Public Health*, 47. Supplement: 4-24 (1957).

B.P. Dohrenwend and B.S. Dohrenwend, *Social Status and Psychological Disorder: A Causal Inquiry* (New York: Wiley-Interscience, 1969).

J.T. Doyle, "Etiology of Coronary Disease: Risk Factors Influencing Coronary Disease," *Mod. Conc. Cardiovascular Dis.*, 35 (1966), pp. 81-86.

F. Dunbar, *Emotions and Body Changes* (New York: Columbia University Press, 1954).

F. Dunbar, *Mind and Body: Psychosomatic Medicine* (New York: Random House, 1948).

B. Farber, "Family Organization and Crisis. Maintenance of Integration in Families with a Severely Mentally Retarded Child," *Monographs of the Society for Research in Child Development*, 25, Serial No. 75 (1960).

V. Francis, B.M. Korsch and M.J. Morris, "Gaps in Doctor-Patient Communication: Patients' Response to Medical Advice," *New England Journal of Medicine*, 280 (1969), pp. 535-540.

C.W. Frank, E. Weinblatt, S. Shapiro and R.V. Sager, "Myocardial Infarction in Men," *Journal of the American Medical Association*, 198,12 (December 1966), pp. 1241-1245.

C.W. Frank, E. Weinblatt, S. Shapiro, G.E. Seiden and R.V. Sager, "The HIP Study of Incidence and Prognosis of Coronary Heart Disease: Criteria for Diagnosis," *Journal of Chronic Diseases*, 16 (1963), pp. 1293-1312.

H.E. Freeman and O. Simmons, *The Mental Patient Comes Home* (New York: Wiley, 1963).

C.L. Friedberg, *Diseases of the Heart* (Philadelphia: W.B. Saunders Company, 3rd edition, 1966).

E.A. Friedman and R.J. Havighurst, *The Meaning of Work and Retirement* (Chicago: University of Chicago Press, 1954).

E.H. Friedman, H.K. Hellerstein, G.L. Eastwood and S.E. Jones, "Behavior Patterns and Serum Cholesterol in Two Groups of Normal Males," *American Journal of the Medical Sciences*, 255 (April 1968), pp. 237-244.

M. Friedman and R.H. Rosenman, *Type A Behavior and Your Heart* (New York: Knopf, 1974).

T. F. Garrity, "Social Involvement and Activeness as Predictors of

Morale Six Months After First Myocardial Infarction," *Social Science and Medicine*, 7 (1973), pp. 199-207.

N. Glazer and D.P. Moynihan, *Beyond the Melting Pot* (Cambridge, Massachusetts: MIT Press, 1963).

T. Gordon, P. Sorlie and W.B. Kannel, "Coronary Heart Disease, Atherothrombotic Brain Infarction, Intermittent Claudication—A Multivariate Analysis of Some Factors Related to Incidence: Framingham Study. 16-Year Follow-up," in W.B. Kannel and T. Gordon (eds.), *The Framingham Study, An Epidemiological Investigation of Cardiovascular Disease* (Washington, D.C.: U.S. Government Printing Office, 1971).

S. Graham and L.G. Reeder, "Social Factors in the Chronic Diseases," in E. Freeman, S. Levine and L.G. Reeder (eds.), *Handbook of Medical Sociology* (Englewood Cliffs: Prentice-Hall, 1972), pp. 63-107.

A.W. Green, "Sexual Activity and the Postmyocardial Infarction," *American Heart Journal*, 89 (February 1975), pp. 246-252.

T.P. Hackett and Ned H. Cassem, "Psychological Adaptation to Convalescence in Myocardial Infarction Patients," in J. Naughton and H.K. Hellerstein (eds.), *Exercise Testing and Exercise Training in Coronary Heart Disease* (New York: Academic Press, 1973).

T.P. Hackett and N.H. Cassem, "Psychological Management of the Myocardial Infarction Patient," *Journal of Human Stress*, 1 (1975), pp. 25-38.

T.P. Hackett and A.D. Weisman, "Denial as a Factor in Patients with Heart Disease and Cancer," *Annals New York Academy of Sciences*, 164 (December 1969), pp. 802-817.

E.C. Hammond and L. Garfinkel, "The Influence of Health on Smoking Habits," *National Cancer Institute, Monograph 19* (1963), pp. 269–285.

E.C. Hammond and L. Garfinkel, "Smoking Habits of Men and Women," *Journal of the National Cancer Institute*, 27 (August 1961), pp 419–421, 426.

D.R. Hay and S. Turbott, "Changes in Smoking Habits in Men Under 65 Years After Myocardial Infarction and Coronary Insufficiency," *British Heart Journal*, 32 (1970), pp. 738-740.

H.K. Hellerstein and E.H. Friedman, "Sexual Activity and the Post-Coronary Patient," *Archives of Internal Medicine*, 125 (1970), pp. 987-999.

H.K. Hellerstein, E. Friedman, P.J. Brdar, M. Weiss, C.W. Dupertuis, D.J. Turell and D. Rumbaugh, "A Comparison of the Personality of Adult Subjects with Rheumatic Heart Disease and With

Arteriosclerotic Heart Disease," Proceedings of Symposium organized by the Council of Rehabilitation of the International Society of Cardiology (Brussels, Belgium, June 1969) pp. 220-282.

G.A. Hellmuth, G. Rodey, W.J. Johannsen and E.L. Belknap, "Work and Heart Disease in Wisconsin," *The Journal of the American Medical Association*, 198 (1966), pp. 9-15.

G.M. Hochbaum, *Public Participation in Medical Screening Programs: A Sociopsychological Study*, (Washington: Public Health Service, Public Health Service Publication No. 572, United States Government Printing Office, 1958).

L. Holder, "Effects of Source, Message, Audience Characteristics on Health Behavior Compliance," *Health Services Reports*, 87 (1972), pp. 343-350.

A.B. Hollingshead, *Two Factor Index of Social Position* (New Haven, Conn.: privately printed, 1957).

A.B. Hollingshead and F.C. Redlich, *Social Class and Mental Illness* (New York: Wiley, 1959).

T.H. Holmes, N.G. Hawkins, C.E. Bowerman, E. Clark, Jr. and J.R. Jaffee, "Psychosocial and Psychophysiologic Studies of Tuberculosis," *Psychosomatic Medicine*, 19 (March-April 1957), pp. 134-143.

M.A. Ibrahim, C.D. Jenkins, J.C. Cassel, J.R. McDonough and C.G. Hames, "Personality Traits and Coronary Heart Disease: Utilization of a Cross-sectional Study Design to Test Whether a Selected Psychological Profile Precedes or Follows Manifest Coronary Heart Disease," *Journal of Chronic Diseases*, 19 (1966), pp. 255-271.

M.A. Ibrahim, D.L. Sackett and S. Kantor, "Psychological Patterns and Coronary Heart Disease: An Appraisal of the Determination of Etiology by Means of a Stochastic Process," *Journal of Chronic Diseases*, 20 (1967), pp. 931-940.

R.K. Idelson, S.H. Croog and S. Levine, "Changes in Self-Concept During the Year After a First Heart Attack: A Natural History Approach," *American Archives of Rehabilitation Therapy*, 22, 1 (March 1974), pp. 10-21; and 22, 2 (June 1974), pp. 25-31.

J.B. Imboden, "Psychosocial Determinants of Recovery," *Advances in Psychosomatic Medicine*, 8 (1972), pp. 142-155.

C.D. Jenkins, "Psychologic and Social Precursors of Coronary Disease," *New England Journal of Medicine*, 284 (1971), pp. 244-255; 307-317.

C.D. Jenkins, R.H. Rosenman and S.J. Zyzanski, "Prediction of Clinical Coronary Heart Disease by a Test for the Coronary-Prone Behavior Pattern," *New England Journal of Medicine*, 290 (1974), pp. 1271-1275.

C.D. Jenkins, S.J. Zyzanski and R.H. Rosenman, "Progress Toward Validation of a Computer-Scored Test for the Type A Coronary-Prone Behavior Pattern," *Psychosomatic Medicine*, 33 (1971), pp. 193-202.

W.J. Johannsen, G.A. Hellmuth and T. Sorauf, "On Accepting Medical Recommendations—Experiences with Patients in a Cardiac Work Classification Unit," *Archives of Environmental Health*, 12 (January, 1966), pp. 63-69.

W.L. Johnson, "Longitudinal Study of Family Adjustment to Myocardial Infarction," *Nursing Research*, Fall Volume (1963), pp. 242-247 (A methodological note).

W.L. Johnson, "A Study of Family Adjustment to the Crisis of Cardiac Disease" (Unpublished manuscript, New York: American Nurses Foundation Inc., 1966).

C. Kadushin, "Social Class and Ill Health: The Need for Further Research," *Sociological Inquiry*, 37 (1967), pp. 323-332.

W.B. Kannel, "Habitual Level of Physical Activity and Risk of Coronary Heart Disease: The Framingham Study," *Canadian Medical Association Journal*, 96 (March 1967), pp. 811-812.

W.B. Kannel, W.P. Castelli and P.M. McNamara, "The Coronary Profile: Twelve-Year Follow-up in the Framingham Study," *Journal of Occupational Medicine*, 9 (1967), pp. 611-619.

W.B. Kannel and M. Feinleib, "Natural History of Angina Pectoris in the Framingham Study. Prognosis and Survival," *American Journal of Cardiology*, 29 (1972), pp. 154-163.

S.V. Kasl, "Issues in Patient Adherence to Health Care Regimens," *Journal of Human Stress*, 1 (1975), pp. 5-17.

S. Kasl and S. Cobb, "Health Behavior, Illness Behavior, and Sick Role Behavior," *Archives of Environmental Health*, 12 (February, 1966), pp. 246-266.

S.S. Kegeles, "Attitudes and Behavior of the Public Regarding Cervical Cytology: Current Findings and New Directions for Research," *Journal of Chronic Diseases*, 20 (1967), pp. 911-922.

S.S. Kegeles, "A Field Experimental Attempt to Change Beliefs and Behavior of Women in an Urban Ghetto," *Journal of Health and Social Behavior*, 10 (1969), pp. 115-125.

S.S. Kegeles, "Why People Seek Dental Care: A Test of a Conceptual Formulation," *Journal of Health and Human Behavior*, 4 (1963), pp. 166-173.

S.S. Kegeles, J.P. Kirscht, D.P. Haefner and I.M. Rosenstock, "Survey of Beliefs About Cancer Detection and Taking Papanicolaou Tests," *Public Health Reports*, 80 (1965), pp. 815-823.

R.A. Keith, B. Lown and F.J. Stare, "Coronary Heart Disease and Behavior Patterns," *Psychosomatic Medicine*, 27 (1965), pp. 424-434.

D. Kenigsberg, S.J. Zyzanski, C.D. Jenkins, W.I. Wardwell and A.T. Licciardello, "The Coronary-Prone Behavior Pattern in Hospitalized Patients With and Without Coronary Heart Disease," *Psychosomatic Medicine*, 36 (1974), pp. 344-351.

F.N. Kerlinger, "Factor Analysis," in *Foundations of Behavior Research* (New York: Holt, Rinehart and Winston, 1964), pp. 650-687.

J.P. Kirscht, "The Health Belief Model and Illness Behavior," *Health Education Monographs*, 2 (1974), pp. 387-407.

H.F. Klarman, "Socioeconomic Impact of Heart Disease," Second National Conference on Cardio-vascular Diseases, *The Heart and Circulation*, v. 2 (Washington, D.C.: Federation of American Societies for Experimental Biology, 1965), pp. 693-707.

R.F. Klein, A. Dean and M.D. Bogdonoff, "The Impact of Illness Upon the Spouse," *Journal of Chronic Disease*, 20 (1967), pp. 241-248.

B.M. Korsch, E.K. Gozzi and V. Francis, "Gaps in Doctor-Patient Communication: Doctor-Patient Interaction and Patient Satisfaction," *Pediatrics*, 42 (1968), pp. 855-871.

M. Koslowsky, S.H. Croog and L. LaVoie, "Perceptions of Etiology in Heart Disease," Mimeo (1977).

T.S. Langner and S.T. Michael, "Life Stress and Mental Health: the Midtown Manhattan Study," A.C. Rennie Series in *Social Psychiatry*, Vol. II (New York: The Free Press, 1963).

P.R. Lee, H. Rusk, P.D. White and B. Williams, "Cardiac Rehabilitation: Questionnaire Survey of Medical Directors in Industry," *Journal of the American Medical Association*, 165 (1957), pp. 787-791.

A.H. Leighton, *My Name Is Legion* (New York: Basic Books, Inc., 1959).

S. Levine and N.A. Scotch, *Social Stress* (Chicago: Aldine, 1970).

E. Lind and T. Theorell, "Sociological Characteristics and Myocardial Infarctions," *Journal of Psychosomatic Research*, 17 (1973), pp. 59-73.

D.T. Linehan, "What Does the Patient Want to Know?" *American Journal of Nursing*, 66 (May 1966), pp. 1066-1070.

R. Linton, "The Natural History of the Family," in R.N. Anshen (ed.), *The Family: Its Function and Destiny* (New York: Harper and Row, 1949), pp. 18-38.

E. Litwak, "Geographic Mobility and Extended Family Cohesion," *American Sociological Review*, 25 (1960), pp. 385-394.

E. Litwak and I. Szelenyi, "Primary Group Structures and Their Functions: Kin, Neighbors, and Friends," *American Sociological Review*, 34 (1969), pp. 465-481.

J. Lorber, "Good Patients and Problem Patients: Conformity and Deviance in a General Hospital," *Journal of Health and Social Behavior*, 16 (1975), pp. 213-225.

M. Marston, "Compliance with Medical Regimens: A Review of the Literature," *Nursing Research*, 19 (1970), pp. 312-323.

A.M. Master, "The Role of Effort and Occupation (Including Physicians) in Coronary Occlusion," *Journal of the American Medical Association*, 174 (1960), p. 942-948.

A.M. Master and S. Dack, "Rehabilitation Following Acute Coronary Occlusion," *Journal of the American Medical Association*, 115 (1940) pp. 828-832.

A.M. Master, H.L. Jaffe, E.M. Teich and L.B. Brinberg, "Survival and Rehabilitation After Coronary Occlusion," *Journal of the American Medical Association*, 156 (1954), pp. 1552-1556.

D. Mechanic, *Medical Sociology, A Selective View* (New York: The Free Press, 1968).

J.H. Medalle, H.A. Kahn, H.N. Neufeld, F. Riss, U. Goldbourt, T. Perlstein, and D. Oron, "Myocardial Infarction Over a Five-Year Period: I. Prevalence, Incidence and Mortality Experience," *Journal of Chronic Diseases*, 26 (1973), pp. 63-84.

H.H.W. Miles, S. Waldfogel, E.L. Barrabee and S. Cobb, "Psychosomatic Study of 46 Young Men With Coronary Artery Disease," *Psychosomatic Medicine*, 16 (1954), p. 455-477.

S. Minc, G. Sinclair and R. Taft, "Some Psychological Factors in Coronary Heart Disease," *Psychosomatic Medicine*, 25 (1963), p. 133-139.

J.H. Mitchell, "Compliance With Medical Regimens: An Annotated Bibliography," *Health Education Monographs*, 2, No. 1 (1974), pp. 75-87.

L.A. Monteiro, "After Heart Attack: Behavioral Expectations for the Cardiac," *Social Science and Medicine*, 7 (1973), pp. 555-565.

A.M. Mordkoff and O.A. Parsons, "The Coronary Personality: A Critique," *Psychosomatic Medicine*, 29 (1967), pp. 1-14.

1. Moriyama, D. Krueger and J. Stamler, *Cardiovascular Diseases in the United States* (Cambridge, Mass.: Harvard University Press, 1971).

J.N. Morris, "Occupation and Coronary Heart Disease," *Archives of Internal Medicine*, 104 (1959) pp. 903-907.

N.C. Morse and R.S. Weiss, "The Function and Meaning of Work and the Job," *American Sociological Review*, 68 (1962), pp. 79-87.

S.J. Mushkin and F. d'A. Collings, "Economic Costs of Disease and Injury," *Public Health Reports*, 74 (1959), pp. 795-809.

J.K. Myers and L.L. Bean, *A Decade Later, A Follow-up of Social Class and Mental Illness* (New York: John Wiley and Sons, Inc., 1968).

J.K. Myers, J.J. Lindenthal, M.P. Pepper and D.R. Ostrander, "Life Events and Mental Status: A Longitudinal Study," *Journal of Health and Social Behavior*, 13 (1972), pp. 398-406.

S. Nagi, *Disability and Rehabilitation* (Columbus: Ohio State University Press, 1969).

National Heart and Lung Institute. Task Force on Cardiovascular Rehabilitation. Needs and Opportunities for Rehabilitating the Coronary Heart Disease Patient. U.S. Government Printing Office. DHEW Pub. No. (NIH) 75-750 (December 1974).

J. Naughton and J. Bruhn, "Emotional Stress, Physical Activity and Ischemic Heart Disease," *DM/Disease-A-Month* (July 1970).

J.P. Naughton and H.K. Hellerstein, *Exercise Testing and Exercise Training in Coronary Heart Disease* (New York: Academic Press, 1973).

J.M. Nunnally, *Psychometric Theory* (New York: McGraw-Hill, 1967).

W.F. Ogburn, "The Family and Its Functions, Recent Social Trends, Report of the President's Research Committee on Social Trends" (New York: McGraw-Hill Book Co., 1934), pp. 661-708.

S. Olshansky, S. Friedland, R.J. Clark and H.B. Sprague, "A Survey of Employment Policies as Related to Cardiac Patients in Greater Boston," *New England Journal of Medicine*, 253 (1955), pp. 506-510.

A.M. Ostfeld, "The Interaction of Biological and Social Variables in Cardiovascular Disease," *Milbank Memorial Fund Quarterly*, 45: Supplement 13-8 (April 1967).

A.M. Ostfeld, B.Z. Lebovits, R.B. Shekelle and O. Paul, "A Prospective Study of the Relationship Between Personality and Coronary Heart Disease," *Journal of Chronic Diseases*, 17 (1964), pp. 265-276.

Howard J. Parad (ed.), *Crisis Intervention: Selected Readings* (New York:

Family Service Association of America, 1965).

Talcott Parsons, "The Kinship System of the Contemporary United States," *American Anthropologist*, 45 (1943), pp. 22-38.

Talcott Parsons and R. Bales, *Family, Socialization, and Interaction Process* (Glencoe, Illinois: Free Press, 1955).

Benjamin Pasamanick, Frank R. Scharpitti and Simon Dinitz, *Schizophrenics in the Community* (New York: Appleton-Century-Crofts, 1967).

H.E.S. Pearson and J. Joseph, "Stress and Occlusive Coronary-Artery Disease," *Lancet*, 1 (1963), pp. 415-418.

A.A.F. Peel, T. Semple, I. Wang, W.M. Lancaster and J.L.G. Dall, "A Coronary Prognostic Index for Grading the Severity of Infarction," *British Heart Journal*, 24, 6 (November, 1972), pp. 745-760.

S. Pell and C.A. D'Alonzo, "Acute Myocardial Infarction in a Large Industrial Population. Report of a 6-Year Study of 1,356 Cases," *Journal of the American Medical Association*, 185 (1963), pp. 831-838.

S. Pell and C.A. D'Alonzo, "Immediate Mortality and Five-Year Survival of Employed Men With a First Myocardial Infarction," *New England Journal of Medicine*, 270 (1964), pp. 915-922.

C.A. Pinderhughes, F.B. Grace, L.J. Reyna and R.T. Anderson," Interrelationships between Sexual Functioning and Medical Conditions," *Medical Aspects of Human Sexuality*, 6 (October 1972), pp. 52-76.

P. Pineo, "Disenchantment in the Later Years of Marriage," *Marriage and Family Living*, 23 (1961), pp. 3-11.

I.B. Pless, K. Roghmann and R.J. Haggerty, "Chronic Illness, Family Functioning, and Psychological Adjustment: A Model for the Allocation of Preventive Mental Health Services," *International Journal of Epidemiology*, 1 (1972), pp. 271-277.

Steven Polgar, "Health Action in Cross-Cultural Perspective," in H.E. Freeman, S.Levine and L.G. Reeder (eds.), *Handbook of Medical Sociology* (Englewood Cliffs, New Jersey: Prentice-Hall, 1972).

L. Pratt, *Family Structure and Effective Health Behavior: The Energized Family* (Boston: Houghton Mifflin, 1976).

E.L. Quarantelli, "A Note on the Protective Function of the Family in Disasters," *Marriage and Family Living*, 22 (1960), pp. 263-264.

R.H. Rahe, "Life Crisis and Health Change," in P.R.A. May and J.R. Wittenborn (eds.), *Psychotropic Drug Response: Advances in Prediction* (Springfield, Illinois: Charles C. Thomas, 1969), p. 92.

R.H. Rahe, D. McKean, Jr. and R.J. Arthur, "A Longitudinal Study of Life: Change and Illness Patterns," *Journal of Psychosomatic Research*, 10 (May, 1967), pp. 355-366.

R. Rapoport, "Normal Crises, Family Structure, and Mental Health," *Family Process*, 2 (1963), pp. 68-80.

G.G. Reader, "The Physician as Teacher," *Health Education Monographs*, 2, No. 1 (1974), pp. 34-38.

L.G. Reeder, "The Socio-Economic Effects of Heart Disease," *Social Problems*, 4 (1956), pp. 51-54.

L.G. Reeder and G.A. Donohue, "Cardiac Employment Potential in Urban Society," *Journal of Chronic Diseases*, 8 (1958), pp. 230-243.

L.G. Reeder, "Employment Practices and the Cardiac," *Journal of Chronic Diseases*, 18 (1965), pp. 951-963.

L.G. Reeder, P.G.M. Shrama and J.M. Dirken, "Stress and Cardiovascular Health: An International Cooperative Study-II The Male Population of a Factory at Zurich," *Social Science and Medicine*, 7 (1973), pp. 585-603.

Dorothy P. Rice, *Economic Costs of Cardiovascular Diseases and Cancer, 1962* (Washington, D.C.: U.S. Government Printing Office, Report Health Economics Series No. 5, DHEW, 1965).

Dorothy P. Rice, *Estimating the Cost of Illness* (Washington, D.C.: U.S. Government Printing Office, Health Economics Series No. 6, 1966).

S.S. Rogers and I.C. Mohler, *Cardiovascular Disease; Epidemiology, Prevention, and Rehabilitation; A Guide to Literature* (New York: IFI/Plenum, 1974).

S.G. Rosenberg, "A Case for Patient Education," *Hospital Formulary Management*, 6 (June 1971), pp. 1-4.

R.H. Rosenman, M. Friedman, C.D. Jenkins and R.W. Bortner, "Is there a Coronary-Prone Personality?" *International Journal of Psychiatry*, 5 (May 1968), pp. 427-429.

R.H. Rosenman, M. Friedman, R. Straus, C.D. Jenkins, S.J. Zyzanski and M. Wurm, "Coronary Heart Disease in the Western Collaborative Group Study. A Follow-up Experience of 4½ Years," *Journal of Chronic Diseases*, 23 (1970) pp. 173-190.

I.M. Rosenstock, "What Research in Motivation Suggests for Public Health," *American Journal of Public Health*, 50 (1960), pp. 295-302.

I.M. Rosenstock, "Why People Use Health Services," *Milbank Memorial Fund Quarterly*, 44 (1966), pp. 94-127.

I. Rosow, *Social Integration of the Aged* (New York: Free Press, 1967).

H.I. Russek and B.L. Zohman, "Relative Significance of Heredity,

Diet, and Occupational Stress in Coronary Heart Disease of Young Adults," *American Journal of Medical Science*, 235 (1958), pp. 266-277.

C. Safilios-Rothschild, *The Sociology and Social Psychology of Disability and Rehabilitation* (New York: Random House, 1970).

H. Sanne, "Exercise Tolerance and Physical Training of Non-Selected Patients After Myocardial Infarction," *Acta Medica Scandinavica Supplementum*, 551 (1973) pp. 1-24.

M. Schar, L.G. Reeder and J.M. Dirken, "Stress and Cardiovascular Health: An International Cooperative Study-I", *Social Science and Medicine*, 7 (1973), pp. 573-584.

J. Schiffman, "Survival Following Certain Cardiovascular Events," Section 25 in W.B. Kannel and T. Gordon (eds.), *The Framingham Study. An Epidemiological Investigation of Cardiovascular Disease* (U.S. Government Printing Office, 1970).

E. Shanas, "Family Help Patterns and Social Class in Three Countries," *Journal of Marriage and the Family*, 29 (1967), pp. 257-266.

S. Shapiro, E. Weinblatt and C.W. Frank, "Return to Work after First Myocardial Infarction," *Archives of Environmental Health*, 24 (January 1972), pp. 17-26.

S. Shapiro, E. Weinblatt, C.W. Frank and R.V. Sager, "The H.I.P. Study of Incidence and Prognosis of Coronary Heart Disease. Preliminary Findings on Incidence of Myocardial Infarction and Angina," *Journal of Chronic Diseases*, 18 (1965), pp. 527-558.

S. Shapiro, E. Weinblatt, C.W. Frank and R.V. Sager. "Incidence of Coronary Heart Disease in a Population Insured for Medical Care (HIP). Myocardial Infarction, Angina Pectoris, and Possible Myocardial Infarction," *American Journal of Public Health*, 59 (Supplement to June 1969), pp. 1-101.

S. Shapiro, E. Weinblatt, C.W. Frank and R.V. Sager, "Social Factors in the Prognosis of Men Following First Myocardial Infarction," *Milbank Memorial Fund Quarterly*, 48 (1970), pp. 37-50.

D.E. Sharland, "Ability of Men to Return to Work After Cardiac Infarction," *British Medical Journal*, 5411, 718 (1964).

R.B. Shekelle, A.M. Ostfeld, B.Z. Lebovits and O. Paul, "Personality Traits and Coronary Heart Disease: A Re-examination of Ibrahim's Hypothesis Using Longitudinal Data," *Journal of Chronic Diseases*, 23 (1970), pp. 33-38.

R.B. Shekelle, A.M. Ostfeld and O. Paul, "Social Status and Incidence of Coronary Heart Disease," *Journal of Chronic Diseases*, 22 (December 1969), pp. 381-394.

D.W. Simborg, "The Status of Risk Factors and Coronary Heart Disease," *Journal of Chronic Diseases*, 22 (February 1970), pp. 515-552.

O.G. Simmons, *Work and Mental Illness: Eight Case Studies* (New York: Wiley, 1965).

R.Smith and A. Lilienfeld, *The OASDI Disability Program. An Evaluation Study*, Final Report (1969).

H.B. Sprague, "Emotional Stress and the Etiology of Coronary Artery Disease," *Circulation*, 17 (1958) pp. 1-4.

J. Stamler, H.A. Lindberg, D.M. Berkson, A. Shaffer, W. Miller and A. Poindexter, "Prevalence and Incidence of Coronary Heart Disease in Strata of the Labor Force of a Chicago Industrial Corporation," *Journal of Chronic Diseases*, 11 (1960), pp. 405-420.

R. Strauss, "Social Change and the Rehabilitation Concept," in M.B. Sussman (ed.), *Sociology and Rehabilitation* (Washington, D.C.: American Sociological Association, 1966).

M.B. Sussman, "Readjustment and Rehabilitation of Patients," in J. Kosa et al. (eds.), *Poverty and Health: A Sociological Analysis* (Cambridge: Harvard University Press, 1969).

M.B. Sussman, "Relationships of Adult Children with Their Parents in the United States," in E.Shanas and G.F. Streib (eds.), *Social Structure and the Family: Generational Relations* (Englewood Cliffs, New Jersey: Prentice-Hall, 1965), pp. 62-92.

M.B. Sussman and L. Burchinal, "Kin Family Network: Unheralded Structure in Current Conceptualizations of Family Functioning," *Marriage and Family Living*, 24 (1962), pp. 231-240.

M.B. Sussman and L. Burchinal, "Parental Aid to Married Children: Implications for Family Functioning," *Marriage and Family Living*, 24 (1962), pp. 320-332.

S.L. Syme, "Social and Psychological Risk Factors in Coronary Heart Disease," *Modern Concepts of Cardiovascular Disease*, 44, 4 (1975), pp. 17-21.

L.S. Syme, H.M. Merton and P.E. Enterline, "Some Social and Cultural Factors Associated With the Occurrence of Coronary Heart Disease," *Journal of Chronic Diseases*, 17 (March 1964), pp. 277-289.

T. Theorell and R.H. Rahe, "Life Change Events, Ballistocardiography and Coronary Death," *Journal of Human Stress*, 1 (1975), pp. 18-24.

R. Treitel, *Rehabilitation of the Disabled*. Social Security Survey of the Disabled: 1966, Report No. 12 (September 1970).

United States Department of Health, Education and Welfare, Public

Health Service, National Institutes of Health. Arteriosclerosis: Report by the National Heart and Lung Institute Task Force on Arteriosclerosis. Vol. 1. (Washington, D.C.: U.S. Government Printing Office, DHEW Pub. No. (NIH) 72-137, June 1971).

R. Useem, J. Useem and D.L. Gibson, "The Function of Neighboring for the Middle Class Male," *Human Organization,* 19 (1960), pp. 68-76.

P. Vincent, "Factors Influencing Patient Noncompliance: A Theoretical Approach," *Nursing Research,* 20 (1971), pp. 509-516.

H. Waitzkin and J.D. Stoeckle, "The Communication of Information About Illness," *Advances in Psychosomatic Medicine,* 8 (1972), pp. 180-215.

W.I. Wardwell and C.B. Bahnson, "Behavioral Variables and Myocardial Infarction in the Southeastern Connecticut Heart Study," *Journal of Chronic Diseases,* 22 (1973), pp. 447-461.

W.I. Wardwell, C.B. Bahnson and H.S. Caron, "Social and Psychological Factors in Coronary Heart Disease," *Journal of Health and Human Behavior,* 4 (1963), pp. 154-185.

L.J. Warshaw, "Putting the Patient with Cardiac Disease Back to Work," *Archives of Environmental Health,* 12 (1966), pp. 651-654.

E. Weinblatt, S. Shapiro and C.W. Frank, "Prognosis of Women With Newly Diagnosed Coronary Heart Disease—A Comparison With Course of Disease Among Men," *American Journal of Public Health,* 63 (July 1973), pp. 577-593.

E. Weinblatt, S. Shapiro, C.W. Frank and R.V. Sager, "Prognosis of Men After First Myocardial Infarction: Mortality and First Recurrence in Relation to Selected Parameters," *American Journal of Public Health,* 58 (1968) pp. 1329-1347.

E. Weinblatt, S. Shapiro and C.W. Frank, "Changes in Personal Characteristics of Men, Over Five Years, Following First Diagnosis of Coronary Heart Disease," *American Journal of Public Health,* 61 (1971), pp. 831-842.

E. Weinblatt, S. Shapiro, C.W. Frank and R.V. Sager, "Return to Work and Work Status Following First Myocardial Infarction," *American Journal of Public Health,* 56 (1966), pp. 169-185.

E. Weiss, B. Dlin, H.R. Rollin, H.K. Fischer and C.R. Bepler, "Emotional Factors in Coronary Occlusion," *Archives of Internal Medicine,* 99 (1957), pp. 628-641.

N. Wenger, "The Early Ambulation of Patients After Myocardial Infarction," *Cardiology,* 58 (1973) pp. 1-6.

N.K. Wenger, C.A. Gilbert and W. Siegel, "Symposium: The Use of

Physical Activity in the Rehabilitation of Patients After Myocardial Infarction," *Southern Medical Journal,* 63 (1970), pp. 891-897.

L. Werko, "Can We Prevent Heart Disease?" *Annals of Internal Medicine,* 74 (1971), pp. 278-288.

L. Werko, "Risk Factors and Coronary Heart Disease—Facts or Fancy?" *American Heart Journal,* 91 (1976), pp. 87-98.

W.F. Whyte, *Men at Work* (Homewood, Illinois: The Dorsey Press, Inc. and Richard D. Irwin, Inc., 1961).

R.F. Winch and S.A. Greer, "Urbanism, Ethnicity, and Extended Familism," *Journal of Marriage and the Family,* 30 (1968), pp. 40-45.

C. Zimmerman and L. Cervantes, *Successful American Families* (New York: Pageant Press, 1960).

B.L. Zohman, "Emotional Factors in Coronary Disease," *Geriatrics* (February 1973), pp. 110-119.

L.R. Zohman and J.S. Tobis, *Cardiac Rehabilitation* (New York: Grune and Stratton, 1970).

W.J. Zukel, R.H. Lewis, P.E. Enterline, R.C. Painter, L.S. Ralston, R.M. Fawcett, A.P. Meredith and B. Peterson, "A Short-term Community Study of the Epidemiology of Coronary Heart Disease," *American Journal of Public Health,* 49 (1959), pp. 1630-1639.

S.J. Zyzanski and C.D. Jenkins, "Basic Dimensions Within the Coronary-Prone Behavior Pattern," *Journal of Chronic Diseases,* 22 (1970), pp. 781-795.

Author Index

Subject Index

Mortality
primary indices of, 306,
307, 309-311, 399, 400
associations with other
outcome indices,
336-338
relationships with an-
tecedent variables,
313 320, 332 335
rating of, rationale for
multi-item-system, 51,
52, 304, 305, 350, 351
secondary indices of, 307-
309, 320-328, 400
associations with other
outcome indices,
336-338
description of, 307-309
relationships with an-
tecedent variables,
322-330, 332-335
See also Heart attack, problems after; Rehabilita-
tion

Patient population, core, 382-388
criteria for selection of, 41,
42, 45, 65, 66, 348, 349,
378, 394-396
See also Data collection;
Methods of research
Patient view of progress, association with other outcome indices, 311, 337
distribution at T_3, 310, 311
as index of outcome, 307,
314, 315
and patient use of health
services, 166
at T_1, as antecedent variable, 325, 327
Pensions, financial assistance

from, 146, 147, 149-151
Personality, and compliance, 201
and work return, 55
Personality self-ratings, of patients, 176, 277-300
change over time, 291-297
and illness level,
297-299
compared with Framing-
ham Heart Study
population, 284-289,
356
and compliance orienta-
tion, 201
and coronary-prone be-
havior pattern (Type A),
176, 275, 283, 356
and denial, 299, 300
factor analysis of, 277,
281-284
and outcome, 331-335
and symptoms at T_3, 352,
353
at T_2, 278-289
See also Denial; Depression;
Anxiety, Self-concept
Physical activity, at work, 101,
102, 107, 116, 117
change in, 116, 117
and depression at T_3, 329,
330
in etiology of heart attack,
107, 108, 122, 123
and occupational level, 116,
117
and outcome, 315, 317,
323, 325, 327, 329, 330,
352
physician advice on, and
occupational level, 171,
172, 184
Physician-patient communication,